The Pocket Diet & Recipe Book
Perfect Portion Control that Works!™

By George Kashou and Caitlyn Lorenze, RD
with Pocket Chef Jenna Bayley-Burke

A LINX Book

Acknowledgements

We would like to thank Community Memorial Hospital, Barb Taggart and her staff of dietitians, and all participants in the Pocket Diet study. We would also like to thank the many people who contributed their ideas during the development of this book.

The Pocket Diet & Recipe Book
©2008 by George Kashou, Kangaroo Brands, Inc.
7620 North 81st Street, Milwaukee, WI 53223
Pocket Diet website: www.pocketdiet.com
All rights reserved. No part of this book may be reproduced
in any form without the prior written permission of the publisher.
ISBN: 0-9802118-0-8
Printed in the United States of America

Book design by Paul Fitzgerald
Contributing writing by Sandra Gurvis

You should always consult with your doctor before making any changes to your diet, or starting an exercise program.

What Registered Dietitians are saying about the Pocket Diet...

"Portion control is the key to achieving & maintaining a healthy weight. This meal plan is designed to teach ideal portion control while eating balanced amounts of nutrients"

> Sharon Yirilli, MS, RD, CDN
> Whitestone, NY

"Simple, satisfying, back to the basics nutrition... that can fit in to anyone's lifestyle"

> Jamie McDermott, MS, RD, CDN
> Bristol, CT

"Great, easy to prepare recipes for on-the-go meals. Perfect for kids, teens & adults"

> Barbara Andresen, RD LDN
> Winston-Salem, NC

"I like that it is comprehensive"

> Cindy Guirino, RD, LD, CNSD
> Dayton, OH

"Easy to follow, encourages use of high fiber foods, very user-friendly portion control"

> Janice Baker, B.Sc., MBA, RD, CDE
> San Diego, CA

"The Pocket Diet offers weight loss with good taste and good nutrition because it doesn't remove foods from your diet. Instead it shows you how much to eat and emphasizes good food choices to reach and maintain a healthier weight"

> Rebecca Schauer, RD, LD
> Minneapolis, MN

"Portion control is the key to achieving & maintaining a healthy weight. This meal plan is designed to teach ideal portion control while eating balanced amounts of nutrients"

Sharon Yirilli, MS RD CDN
Whitestone, NY

"It's a very clever, practical idea. I wish that I thought of it!"

Rebecca Bitzer, MS, RD
Greenbelt, MD

"I think this provides a very easy & user friendly way to control portion size - which is critical to losing weight. The recipes are great"

Dianne Scheinberg
Newton, MA

"The Pocket Diet book provides sound nutrition advice and balanced, healthy meals for all people struggling to lose weight"

Betsy Oriolo, MS, RD,LD, CDE
Burlington KY

"A useful plan to help people moderate portion sizes while at the same time enjoying a wide variety of healthy foods"

Lynn Grieger, RD, LD, CDE
Manchester Center, VT

"This meal plan makes sense and is practical, easy and medically sound"

Kim Slominsky, RD
Bogota NJ

"The teaching of portion sizes is perfect! No measuring is such a plus"

Lisa Corman, RD, LD
Dover, NH

contents

foreword

Donna M. Manning, DTR,
Registered Dietetic Technician

Congratulations on choosing the Pocket Diet. There are many aspects of life that we cannot change. However, you can control your weight and opt to live a healthy lifestyle. It is up to you!

People have different reasons for deciding to adopt healthy eating habits. Whether it's for weight loss, more energy, or to simply live a longer and better life, you'll need to work on certain behaviors and learn new ones.

There are some things you can do to help you succeed. First, set reasonable and obtainable goals. They can be both short and long-term but should be realistic, inspiring you and giving you incentive to stick with the program. Gradual small changes can add up to positive results. It takes time to change behaviors, but anything worth having is worth the effort. So believe in yourself and visualize achieving your goals.

Next, list all the reasons why you have chosen a healthier lifestyle. Some could be to lose weight, look better, live longer, buy new clothes, or whatever comes to mind.

Third, make a list of actions to accomplish your goal. These could be: follow the Pocket Diet plan, walk 20 minutes a day, drink plenty of water, and so on. Include physical activity in this plan. Chooseactivities you enjoy: walking, biking, dancing, gardening, swimming and so on. Vary your activity to keep it fun. Have some workout partners to keep you motivated. All activities, even taking the stairs instead of the elevator, will burn calories. Physical activity is not only good for your health, but it also raises your metabolism and self-esteem. It will make you feel good and help you keep your goals in focus.

Once you finish your list, type it up and place it on your refrigerator or your bathroom mirror. Read the list often and make notes of your progress. These actions will empower and motivate you. Fad diets come and go, but the key elements to controlling your weight for the long term are:

1. Educating your self on proper nutrition.
2. Adopting new habits so you can eat healthy.

These are the most effective ways to control your weight for a lifetime.

I endorse the Pocket Diet because it promotes common sense eating with a variety of great tasting foods. It is convenient to follow, and this makes it sustainable over a long period of time. Perhaps best of all, it teaches portion control, which is key to reducing calories and weight.

Think of food as fuel for your body. How much fuel does your body need so you feel good? Eating healthy is not just about weight loss and maintenance, but also creating balance between calories eaten and calories burned. This is key to controlling your weight. The Pocket Diet will help you to control your portions, calories, and weight.

Eating is one of life's greatest pleasures, and all foods can fit into a healthy lifestyle. One of the exciting things in choosing to be healthy is making choices that are best for you. It is not one size fits all. Discover what works, and make it fun. Life is a journey and you can help create your own destiny and enjoy it more by making healthy choices.

Along with being a dietetic technician (DTR) registered with the American Dietetic Association, Donna M. Manning is a professional motivational speaker in the field of nutrition. They say you are what you eat... so what are you now?

And what do you want to be?

introduction

The Pocket Diet is an effective and convenient plan that uses tasty and nutritious pita pocket bread to teach portion control to help you achieve a healthy weight. This book also provides complete but concise and easy-to-understand information about basic and sound nutrition. It will help you determine how much food to eat based on your body type, understand your metabolism, and empower you to improve your health and control your weight for life.

By simply adopting the basics of portion control taught by the Pocket Diet, excess weight will be shed slowly and permanently. The Pocket Diet is a "back to the basics" approach that will help avoid the up-and-down, yo-yo effect inherent with so many of today's diet plans.

The Pocket Diet will provide you with a smooth transition from your current eating habits to an improved and healthier way of eating. It is convenient to follow and easy to maintain because you are allowed to eat everyday foods and snacks.

Remember that portion control is the key to successful weight control. Ther pocket diet is the only diet plan that offers a convenient, healthy and edible food container -- a wholesome bread product -- that will help control meal portions. Dieting to lose weight is not just about what you eat, but how much. Choosing the right foods is vital to maintaining good health.

Why the Pocket Diet?

The healthcare community knows more than ever about what foods help the human body to be lean, energetic and efficient. More is being discovered each day about the links between obesity and heart disease, cancer, diabetes and other ailments. Yet the public is gaining weight at an alarming rate.

Losing weight has always been tough work. With current on-the-go lifestyles and dual income families, the days of spending long afternoons preparing meals with healthy, fresh foods from the garden and the butcher's are long gone. Family dinners have been replaced with a cell phone call checking in to see who is going to be picking what from which carryout. And the job of portion control has been turned over to restaurants and fast food chains. There is a better way. With the Pocket Diet, you can eat deliciously and nutritiously in spite of today's fast-paced, fast-food lifestyles. This book offers simple and practical tips for lifelong portion control, weight loss, and healthy eating. Much of the information is based on the research from the National Institutes of Health, the American Heart Association, and the Institute of Medicine. But we've put it together so it's easy to follow and will work.

About the Pocket Diet Creators:

George Kashou: Of Mediterranean heritage, George Kashou grew up in a family that practiced good nutrition, long before the topic became mainstream. He, his wife and two adult daughters still dine on this healthy cuisine.

George's idea of exercise and relaxation are one in the same. He enjoys projects that require hard physical labor, such as landscaping and gardening. He maintains, tills and plants a large organic garden that helps to feed five families with plenty of leftovers for co-workers. His idea of recreational heaven on earth is downhill skiing.

A lifelong entrepreneur, George is quick to recognize opportunities and implement ideas. Twenty-five years ago he and his brother John started Kangaroo Brands, Inc. a small bakery. George and John set out to Americanize pita pockets, an ethnic specialty bread with limited distribution. Along with producing a high quality pita pocket that was easy to use, they received a federal patent for the "greatest innovation since sliced bread," a pre-opened pita pocket that is easy to fill without tearing. Today they sell their pita pocket breads -- the #1 brand in Deli – Bakery section in the U.S. -- in over 9,000 retail stores here and in Canada. George is the vice-president of sales and marketing for Kangaroo Brands.

But despite these accomplishments, George felt more needed to be done. He was disturbed by negative influence and lack of safety in fad diets. His believed that such diets preyed on too many people, including members of his extended family and friends. He recognized a need for a sensible approach to weight loss and decided write a book on nutrition. The result can be found in these pages.

Caitlyn E. Lorenze, Registered Dietitian (RD): A lifelong athlete, Caitlyn Lorenze has always understood the role of healthy eating and its relationship to optimal performance. From the field hockey grounds to the triathlon course, she has discovered first hand how the right fuel can make the difference in achieving athletic and health goals.

This awareness and a passion for helping others improve their health through nutrition and fitness sparked her interest in nutrition at the academic level. Caitlyn earned a Bachelor's degree in Dietetics from the University of Maryland. Not losing sight on her link to athletics, Caitlyn also became a certified personal trainer, while simultaneously completing an internship with the American Dietetic Association at Virginia Polytechnic Institute and State University.

In 2003, Caitlyn founded wholesomebody, LLC to help individuals understand the role of nutrition in healthy living. The challenge of running a business, making healthy food choices and finding time for training has made Caitlyn truly appreciate the need for great-tasting, convenient good food, hence her participation in the Pocket Diet. Identifying simple ways to improve diet has become a trademark of her business.

Jenna Bayley-Burke, The Pocket Chef: Jenna lives in the Pacific Northwest, developing award winning recipes from her home kitchen. Her creations have appeared in Better Homes & Gardens, Sunset, Cooking Light, and Cuisine at Home.

She believes in keeping food simple, making sure all of our Pocket Diet recipes could be prepared with a minimum of effort and the least amount of kitchen gadgets. A mother of two, she understands how important it is to get healthy food on the table, fast, while still pleasing the pickiest of palates.

Food should never be boring, so the recipes vary from basic to inspired and everywhere in between. The Pocket Diet can go anywhere, mold into any lifestyle, helping portion control to become second nature.

Jenna is a domestic engineer, romance novelist, cookbook author, freelance writer, recipe developer, and chocolate fanatic. She hides out in the Pacific Northwest with her high school sweetheart and two blueberry eyed baby boys, who all have her wrapped around their little fingers.

Obesity: An American Epidemic

At any given moment, approximately 50 million Americans are searching for the miracle diet -- some kind of fast, safe and easy way to lose weight and improve their health and outlook on life. There appears to be an ever-growing audience awaiting an instant panacea.

According to the Centers for Disease Control (www.cdc.gov) and the Journal of the American Medical Association (JAMA):

- Between the years 1960 and 2000 the number of obese adults in the US doubled.

- Currently 70% of Americans are overweight or obese, and this is a growing epidemic.

- $50 billion is spent annually on quackery diets, supplements and weight-loss devices.

The dieting dilemma is nothing new. "Diet consciousness" can be traced back to an 1869 book, "Letter on Corpulence," which was written by William Banting in London. The book sold for one shilling ($0.88), a miniscule trickle in what was to become a multi-billion dollar diet book industry.

Despite the thousands of diet books written since then, Americans still struggle to discover the Holy Grail of weight loss. As you will learn, the key to lifelong diet success is as simple as balance between sensible eating and maintaining an ongoing fitness program.

one

The Pocket Diet: An Effective Way to Manage Your Weight

What is The Pocket Diet?

The Pocket Diet offers a new twist to portion control:

- It is convenient, easy to follow and automatically teaches portion control through the use of a pita pocket "edible container" holding the right amount of a variety of healthy foods.

- It is based on eating and enjoying well-balanced meals from all food groups.

- It allows for two to three snacks per day to help control hunger.

- It benefits the entire family. There is no need to prepare special meals for those trying to lose weight.

- It offers easy, multiple-serving recipes that can be made in advance, refrigerated and then used as needed to prepare a quick meal.

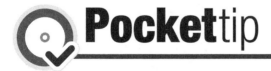

Pockettip

Check with you doctor before beginning a program, especially if you are over 35, obese and/or have not exercised in a long time

Why the Pocket Diet was Created

1. Many diets in today's marketplace are difficult to follow or make unrealistic demands on time-pressed consumers.

2. Pita pockets provide the ideal food container. One pocket bread holds the right portion size for a variety of healthy foods, and it fits the need of today's busy, on-the-go lifestyle.

3. Whole grain products are an integral part of a healthy and balanced diet. As such, learning to properly incorporate them into a weight loss plan can bring about great success.

4. Bread and complex carbohydrates are an important component of the food pyramid. Bread contains fiber, plant proteins, minerals and micronutrients. Carbohydrates are critical to proper brain function and are recommended as a supply of approximately 50% of the body's energy needs.

Pocket Diet Study: Proven Effective and Satisfying

The Pocket Diet was developed in cooperation with Community Memorial Hospital (CMH), in Menomonee Falls, Wisconsin. It was tested with a controlled study group of 38 participants during a six-week period.

Dietitians analyzed the recipes for calories, fat, cholesterol, carbohydrates, sugars, protein and fiber. The flexible meal plans allowed the participants to select the recipe of their choice for any meal. Two meal plans were developed: a 1,500-calorie daily diet for people shorter than 5'6" and an 1,800-calorie for people taller than 5'6".

Participants were at least 15 pounds overweight, had a Body Mass Index (BMI) greater than 25 (BMI will be discussed in Chapter 2), and wanted to lose 1-2 pounds per week. They weighed in weekly. Exercise was encouraged and alcohol consumption was discouraged. All 38 participants completed the study.

Results after Six Weeks:

- The group lost a total of 295 pounds
- The average weight loss was 8 pounds per person
- The greatest weight loss was 18 pounds; the least was 1.5 pounds
- The average weekly loss was 1.3 pounds per person
- The average pocket bread consumption was 4 pockets per day

The following statements were made by the participants at the conclusion of the study:

- "The pocket helped me control my meal portion"
- "The Pocket Diet was the easiest diet I have ever tried"
- "I was happy eating pocket bread on a daily basis"
- "The recipes were easy to prepare"
- "I have recommended this diet to my friends"

A follow-up survey conducted 90 days after the study found that of the 29 dieters who responded, (76% of the original 38) found these results:

- 79% of those surveyed were still following the Pocket Diet
- 73% had gotten closer to their weight loss objectives
- 94% were still using Kangaroo pocket breads as part of their daily diet

These findings suggest that the Pocket Diet is an effective way to lose weight and learn portion control. All of the participants were satisfied with the meal plan and the recipes provided and used the Kangaroo pocket breads to control their food portions. By following the USDA's food pyramid guidelines, the participants' nutritional needs were met as they lost weight.

Testimony: Barb Taggart, Registered Dietitian (RD)
Note: Ms. Taggart is the   Supervisor of Clinical Dietetics at Community Memorial Hospital and she directed the diet study.

Working on the Pocket Diet has been one of my most rewarding projects. It was truly amazing to watch the success of those who followed this program. It's really an instruction in healthy eating and portion control. Like most people, the participants were craving a program that taught them about good nutrition.

In this world of overabundance and fad diets, it has become difficult to know what normal eating really is. The Pocket Diet follows the basic principles of adequate amounts of carbohydrates, reduced fat and increased fiber. You develop a lifelong commitment to healthy eating when you get the right balance of nutrients including carbohydrates and protein. The Pocket Diet does that as well.

The results of the study spoke for itself. All participants lost weight. They embraced the ability of the pocket bread to control their portions. Due to the convenience of the pocket bread, they utilized the plan while on vacation, caring for a sick parent or working full time. One participant, who had been told she would never lose weight due to her health condition, lost 14 pounds in 6 weeks! Perhaps best of all, most participants adopted the Pocket Diet as a way of life. As a registered dietitian, I am confident the Kangaroo Pocket Diet can help bring healthy eating back into focus for you!

Diet and Weight Loss Facts

But there's more to losing weight than following a diet. Dieting to lose weight is determined by how much you eat. Maintaining good health is all about the food you choose to eat. Sometimes these can be at cross-purposes.

Let's start by reviewing the process used to describe a safe, healthy and effective diet that will help you lose weight. Following are some facts about achieving and maintaining the proper weight and a healthy body:

1. You will gain weight if you consume more calories than your body burns off, and lose weight if you burn more calories than you consume.

2. 3,500 calories equals one pound of body weight. This means that if you consume 3,500 calories more than you burn, you will gain one pound. To lose one pound per week a person needs to burn 3,500 calories more per week than he or she consumes.

3. Exercise will increase your metabolism, help you burn calories and strengthen your heart.

4. Water is absolutely essential for health; drink a minimum of six, preferably eight, eight–ounce glasses per day.

5. Dietary fiber, found in natural foods such as whole grains, legumes, fruits and vegetables, is essential for a healthy intestinal tract and can help to improve cholesterol levels in some people.

6. Simple carbohydrates, such as the refined sugar found in convenience food, should be consumed sparingly, because they have little, if any, nutritional value. They only and provide "empty calories."

7. Complex carbohydrates are the body's preferred source of fuel for energy. They also provide fiber, which aids digestion.

8. Protein is essential for healthy body and muscle tissue. Meat, fish, legumes and dairy products are all excellent sources of protein.

9. Fats are essential. The healthiest fats are monounsaturated and polyunsaturated fats, which are found in seeds, nuts, fish oils and liquid vegetable oils. Saturated fats in meats and dairy should be consumed sparingly. Transfats in solid shortenings, margarine, and many sweet baked goods, should be completely avoided.

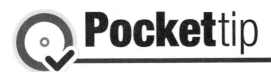

Pockettip

Eat breakfast every day. People who eat breakfast are less likely to overeat later in the day. Breakfast also give you energy and help you keep mentally sharp throughout the day.

Quick Quiz

Ask Yourself the Following 15 Questions:

		YES	NO
1.	Do you eat different colored vegetables daily?	___	___
2.	Do you monitor your daily calorie intake?	___	___
3.	Do you cook more often than not?	___	___
4.	Do you often skip breakfast?	___	___
5.	Do you enjoy deep-fried foods?	___	___
6.	Do you like to eat a lot of food every day?	___	___
7.	Do you enjoy eating convenience food?	___	___
8.	Do you read the nutritional information on the foods you buy?	___	___
9.	Do you follow a regular exercise program?	___	___
10.	Do you frequent fast-food restaurants more than once per week?	___	___
11.	Do you eat bread?	___	___
12.	Do you know the difference between healthy and unhealthy foods?	___	___
13.	Do you know the nutritional value of foods you eat every day?	___	___
14.	Do you believe the expression, "You are what you eat"?	___	___
15.	Do you think will gain more weight by consuming your daily calories from carbs vs. protein and fat?	___	___

(Answers: 1. Y; 2. Y; 3.Y; 4.N; 5. N; 6. N; 7. N; 8.Y; 9.Y; 10.N; 11. Y; 12.Y; 13. Y; 14. Y; 15. N.) If you missed more than 5 questions, the following chapters will hopefully help you get them all right the next time you take the quiz.

Portion Control: An Essential Principle of the Pocket Diet

Most Americans struggle with their weight because they eat too much. The answer to maintaining proper weight is portion control. Because it's a 1.3-ounce, edible food container that holds hot or cold foods, the pita pocket will help you avoid eating too much.

Think of eating the same way as you would as managing your money. If you can manage a financial budget, then you can also learn to handle a caloric budget. First you need to know how many calories you can afford to consume, and second you need to learn the caloric values of foods. Always choose the best nutritional value for the foods selected, within your calorie limit.

In a Pocket: The Basic Pocket Diet Plan

The plan is simple and described below. The key is to choose your foods carefully and get the best nutritional value for the calories you consume.

- Eat 3 meals per day using pita pockets to measure the portion size of your meals (You can choose almost any foods. Just make sure they fit into your pita pocket.)

- Eat 2-3 snacks per day (Designated portions of fruit, nuts, veggies, yogurt or cottage cheese)

- Start and maintain an ongoing fitness program

Remember to ration the servings of the various foods throughout the day, to include three balanced meals plus 2-3 snacks in controlled portions.

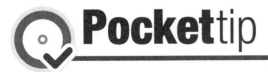

Pockettip

Watch the sugar! Cut back on beverages and foods with added sugars. A 12 oz. can of "regular" soda can have as many as 150 calories!

Pocket Diet Preview

The following illustrates the amount of food you will need to stay within approximately 1,500 calories per day. This sample menu provides a "taste" of what to expect in Chapter 5, which will have a thorough description of the meal plan.

Meal	Food Choices	Approximate Calories
Breakfast:	Egg, ham & cheese in 1 pocket	220
AM Snack:	Low-fat yogurt or fruit	100
Lunch:	Tuna or chicken salad in 2 pockets, and fruit	500
PM Snack:	Fruit, nuts, or raw veggies	130
Dinner:	4-5 oz. of meat or fish 1 serving complex carb + vegetable	450
Evening Snack	Fruit, nuts, yogurt or Reduced-fat ice cream	100

Total Calories: 1,500

Convenience: The Pocket Diet Difference

One wonders why there are so many diets when the principles of safe and healthy weight loss are so basic. People are constantly seeking a "miracle" that will bring quick results without a lot of work.

A diet that requires significant effort may be difficult to sustain and ultimately lead to failure. We are creatures of habit. When asked to make sacrifices or otherwise drastically alter our habits, we rebel and ultimately fail.

That is why it is so important to be realistic when deciding on a diet, whether it is the Pocket Diet or another safe and realistic plan. Convenience, variety and taste are keys to success. Healthy, enjoyable and easy-to-prepare foods need to be available when you're hungry.

When considering a diet, ask yourself the following questions:

- Will my family and I enjoy eating the recommended foods?

- Are the foods easy to prepare?

- Does the diet require any significant extra work for my family and me?

- Is the diet safe and healthy?

Today's dual-income households and on-the-go lifestyles leave little time for meal preparation. The last thing you need is to spend more time and effort fixing special "diet" meals. Along with providing recipes, exercises, and nutrition tips, upcoming chapters will also help you manage your eating and make the best and most convenient choices for your lifestyle.

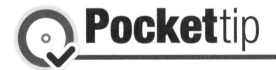

Pockettip

Don't Diet – Change. Ninety five percent of people who diet regain the weight when they stop. It's not only discouraging, but bad for your health. Instead of starting a diet that requires you to alter what, how much and how you eat all at once, make small (but permanent) changes everyday. Ask yourself each morning, "What is one thing I can do today to be healthier?" and then do it. Some goals will stick and others won't, but you'll see progress.

WEIGHT LOSS 101

Metabolism - Your Body's Engine

Metabolism is your body's motor. It processes and burns calories. If your metabolism is idle, your body will burn only the minimum amount of calories necessary to keep the body functioning. However, even a slightly accelerated metabolic rate can be a significant help in burning extra calories.

Three critical elements accelerate or trigger your metabolism to burn calories.

1. Exercise. This is the best way to increase your metabolic rate. See chart on pages (49) showing calories burned for various activity levels.

2. Increase muscle mass. Muscle burns calories. Even when you're inactive, it keeps your metabolism going at a higher rate.

3. Proper eating. When your body consumes food, it must process, or metabolize it. It's like fuel for your car. You must keep it filled up in order for it to run. But unlike your car, when your body is starved, your metabolism slows down to preserve its stored fuel, and therefore burns fewer calories per hour. Consequently, this metabolic slow down is why you should never skip meals. We recommend eating every 3-4 hours to keep your metabolism running at its most efficient speed.

Does Dieting Work?

Calories in food are derived from protein, carbohydrates and fat. Most of the 300+ diets in today's marketplace follow one of the basic principles listed below and are:

•   Low in (saturated) fat for heart problems and reducing cholesterol

- Low glycemic for diabetes (restricting simple sugars or carbohydrates)

- Well-balanced/calorie measured

The Pocket Diet is a well-balanced and heart healthy, calorie-measured diet that follows the new USDA's food pyramid guide. The fiber in whole wheat and whole grain pita pockets contributes to a lower glycemic index compared to many foods. Low-fat fillings help maintain a heart- healthy approach.

Additionally, there are two types of diets:

- Exclusive diets that achieve weight loss by severely restricting what a person eats

- Inclusive diets that offer flexibility and choice, and focus on portion size and nutrition

The Pocket Diet is an inclusive diet. Rather than restricting what you eat, it guides you as to how much you should consume. The food choices are yours to make.

We hope you would choose the healthier foods, because you are what you eat. However, even if you indulge in some less-nutritious "favorites," the portion-control aspect of this diet will still help you lose weight.

Before beginning, you might want to ask yourself: "Am I dieting just to lose weight, or to improve my health?" Hopefully, your answer will be that you're dieting to improve your health – and lose weight in the process.

Body Mass Index: What You Should Weigh

Being overweight can aggravate arthritis or lower back problems and cause diabetes, heart disease and gallbladder disease. Excess weight has also been associated with breast, uterine, ovarian and other cancers. The government has developed a tool to determine your risk based on your weight called the Body Mass Index (BMI). Use the table below to determine your individual risk.

Calculating BMI is simple, quick, and inexpensive — but it does have limitations. One problem with using BMI as a measurement tool is that muscular or large boned people may fall into the "overweight" category when they are actually healthy and fit. Another problem with using BMI is that people who have lost muscle mass, such as the elderly, may be in the "healthy weight" category — according to their BMI — when they actually have reduced nutritional reserves. BMI, therefore, is useful as a general guideline to monitor trends in the population, but by itself is not diagnostic of an individual's health status. Further evaluation should be performed to determine associated health risks.

Body Mass Index Table

To use the table, find the appropriate height in the left-hand column labeled Height. Move across to a given weight. The number at the top of the column is the BMI at that height and weight. Pounds have been rounded off.

BMI	19	20	21	22	23	24	25	26	27	28	29	30	31	32	33	34	35	36	37	38	39	40:
Height (Inches)																						
58	91	96	100	105	110	115	119	124	129	134	138	143	148	153	158	162	167	172	177	181	186	191
59	94	99	104	109	114	119	124	128	133	138	143	148	153	158	163	168	173	178	183	188	193	198
60	97	102	107	112	118	123	128	133	138	143	148	153	158	163	168	174	179	184	189	194	199	204
61	100	106	111	116	122	127	132	137	143	148	153	158	164	169	174	180	185	190	195	201	206	211
62	104	109	115	120	126	131	136	142	147	153	158	164	169	175	180	186	191	196	202	207	213	218
63	107	113	118	124	130	135	141	146	152	158	163	169	175	180	186	191	197	203	208	214	220	225
64	110	116	122	128	134	140	145	151	157	163	169	174	180	186	192	197	204	209	215	221	227	232
65	114	120	126	132	138	144	150	156	162	168	174	180	186	192	198	204	210	216	222	228	234	240
66	118	124	130	136	142	148	155	161	167	173	179	186	192	198	204	210	216	223	229	235	241	247
67	121	127	134	140	146	153	159	166	172	178	185	191	198	204	211	217	223	230	236	242	249	255
68	125	131	138	144	151	158	164	171	177	184	190	197	204	210	216	223	230	236	243	249	256	262
69	128	135	142	149	155	162	169	176	182	189	196	203	210	216	223	230	236	243	250	257	263	270
70	132	139	146	153	160	167	174	181	188	195	202	209	216	222	229	236	243	250	257	264	271	278
71	136	143	150	157	165	172	179	186	193	200	208	215	222	229	236	243	250	257	265	272	279	286
72	140	147	154	162	169	177	184	191	199	206	213	221	228	235	242	250	258	265	272	279	287	294
73	144	151	159	166	174	182	189	197	204	212	219	227	235	242	250	257	265	272	280	288	295	302
74	148	155	163	171	179	186	194	202	210	218	225	233	241	249	256	264	272	280	287	295	303	311
75	152	160	168	176	184	192	200	208	216	224	232	240	248	256	264	272	279	287	295	303	311	319
76	156	164	172	180	189	197	205	213	221	230	238	246	254	263	271	279	287	295	304	312	320	328

Weight (Pounds)

A healthy weight is an index of 19-25, moderately overweight is an index of 26-29, and severely overweight is an index over 30.

Keep in mind this BMI chart does not take into consideration an individual's bone structure or muscle mass. People that are large boned or have more muscle mass may weigh more than this chart shows, but still be in a healthy weight range.

Basal Metabolic Rate: How Much Should You Eat

The answer depends on your current weight, activity level, age, and metabolism, but eating is only one part of the formula.

A sedentary woman burns only 10 calories per pound of body weight while a man burns 11 calories. That means a 150-pound female would burn 1,500 calories per day just to keep her heart beating, lungs breathing and brain functioning. The minimum number of calories your body requires to maintain itself if you were laying down all day and night in a sedentary position (but not sleeping) is referred to as the body's Basal Metabolic Rate (BMR).

Calories burned increase dramatically with physical activity. This is referred to as the AMR, or the Active Metabolic Rate. This determines the number of calories your body burns for its activity level. For example, a lightly active, 150-pound female may burn off 1800 calories per day.

The following information will help you calculate the number of calories you burn in a normal day. In this way, you can determine how many calories you can consume and still lose weight. However, once the weight is lost you should continue being active. In order to maintain your desired weight, you must continually balance your daily intake with your level of activity and the calories your body burns.

Still, we all overeat occasionally. What's important is to make a conscious effort to balance any over-eating with extra activity, or get back on a sensible food portions in subsequent days.

Calorie Chart

Formula: Weight X Multiplier = Calories burned per day
(i.e., The BMR for a woman is: 10 X 150lb. = 1,500 calories
The BMR for a man : 11 X 200 lb. = 2,200 calories)

Activity Level	Woman (multiplier)	Men (multiplier)
BMR- Sedentary:	10	11
Light Activity:	12	13
Moderate Exercise:	13	14
Moderate/Heavy Exercise:	15	16
Regular Heavy Exercise	17	18

For example, a 200-pound man who is sedentary burns 2,200 calories per day (200 x 11). The same man with moderate exercise burns 2,800 calories per day (200 x 14). An average 150 lb. woman who is sedentary burns 1,500 calories per day (150 x 10). With moderate exercise she burns 1,950 calories (150 x 13) which is a 450 calorie difference.

A woman with moderate exercise alone burns an extra 13,500 calories per month. This translates into a weight loss of 4 pounds or 1 pound per week. (450 x 30 days =13,500 divided by 3,500 calories per pound = 4 lbs.).

Managing and Improving Metabolism

Metabolism is the process that converts food to energy. Think of metabolism as the speed at which your body's engine operates. Basal metabolism is the energy you need when your body's engine is idling – when you're in a reclined position. It gives your body the energy it needs to maintain its basic functions and accounts for about 75% of the calories expended daily.

Some people have faster body engines. Because their basal metabolism is higher, they burn off more calories. People with a lower basal metabolism will have a more difficult time burning off calories.

The good news is that there are safe methods to improve your metabolic rate.

Eight Safe and Natural Ways To Rev Up Your Metabolism

1. Always eat breakfast. Skipping breakfast puts the body in a defensive mode. When the body senses it is low on fuel (food), it slows your metabolic rate to conserve energy.

2. Never eat less than 1,200 calories per day. Your body needs a minimum of 1,200 calories daily just to perform its basic functions. Anything less will prompt the body to slow down its processes, including metabolism.

3. Snack on complex carbohydrates. Fruits, vegetables, and grains fuel your metabolism, and have fewer calories per gram than fat (Carbs have 4 calories per gram vs. the 9 calories per gram in fats).

4. Exercise on a daily basis. Daily exercise will improve your metabolism. A brisk 15-30 minute walk after lunch or dinner energizes the body by boosting your heart rate and blood flow.

5. Tone your muscles with weight training. Toned muscles charge your metabolism and muscle naturally burns more calories.

6. Avoid alcohol. Alcohol depresses your metabolism while stimulating appetite.

7. Look for situations to be active. Instead of finding the closest parking spot, park farther away and walk the distance. Use stairs instead of elevators. These small things can significantly increase the amount of exercise you get each day.

8. Stay hydrated. Try to drink a cup of water every few hours, drinking eight or more 8-oz glasses a day. Your body needs plenty of water to function optimally. Carry a bottle of water with you and drink throughout the day.

Water, Water, Everywhere

Water, the most common substance on earth, is also the nutrient that your body needs the most. Between 60-70% of an adult's body weight is water. Water is critical in regulating all organs and body temperature, as well as dissolving solids and carrying nutrients throughout the body.

Dehydration is the loss of water and electrolytes needed for normal body functioning. Staying hydrated is essential to keeping yourself healthy.

Symptoms of dehydration include:

- General fatigue, lightheadedness, dizziness, headaches and nausea

- Muscle fatigue, cramps and a general loss of endurance

- Fainting, in cases of extreme dehydration

Severe dehydration can lower blood pressure, weaken the heart, and shut down the kidneys. One of the best ways to recognize dehydration is to pay close attention to the color of your urine. Ideally, light to clear urine indicates proper water intake. Dark yellow urine may be a sign of dehydration.

The average person should drink 8 eight-ounce glasses of water or other fluids daily. Do not substitute coffee, tea or soda for water. Caffeine in particular acts as a diuretic, pulling water from your body.

Tips For Keeping Yourself Hydrated:

- Drink extra water on hot summer days, or if you stay outdoors for extended periods of time in cold weather. Dehydration occurs more rapidly in extreme temperatures through perspiration and breathing.

- Caffeine, alcohol and tobacco dehydrate the body. Drink equal amounts of water to equal your consumption of alcohol or caffeine.

Weight Loss Tips and Traps

Choosing a weight loss program is almost as important as selecting a career. It can greatly improve your quality of life (or conversely have a negative impact on your health), so evaluate each diet carefully. Weight loss depends on controlling the calories consumed, regular exercise, curtailing convenience food and making a long-term commitment to healthy eating habits.

Follows are five tips for long-term success:

1. Never skip breakfast. Eating breakfast charges your metabolism and gives your body the energy it needs to get through the morning.

2. Drink eight 8-oz. glasses of water or fluids every day.

3. Eat like your ancestors. Your diet should include fruits, vegetables, grains & breads, legumes, lean meats and fish. Avoid convenience and highly processed foods.

4. Eat something nutritious every three to four hours.

5. Stay physically active.

On the other hand, avoid such weight loss "traps" as:

*   You can eat as many low-fat foods as you desire. (zero grams of fat does not equal zero calories)

*   There are different kinds of calories. (All calories are calories)

*   It is possible to lose 50 pounds in 6 weeks, 5 pounds in a weekend, or any number of pounds without exercise. (It is possible, but not healthy. Rapid weight loss is mostly water weight and this can result in dehydration, which is very dangerous and weight is usually quickly regained.

*   You can shed pounds by merely wearing a belt, ring or bracelet. (Yes, and the Brooklyn Bridge is for sale, too!)

Also be very careful with drugs that claim to aid in weight loss. They may have dangerous side effects that may not be immediately noticeable.

Examples of how diets can be easily sabotaged.

- One extra meal at fast food restaurant contains approximately 1500 calories: 700 calories in the sandwich, 540 calories in the French fries and 310 calories in the drink. Add a shake for dessert and you're up to 2,000 calories in just one meal!

- Three slices of pizza and a large soft drink will add about 1,200 calories to your diet.

- Ten creme sandwich cookies will cost you 550 calories, for many one-fourth of their recommended daily caloric intake.

- Beware of snacking. Potato chips, cookies, donuts and candy bars are all convenience foods that are easily consumed in large quantities. Even peanuts, which are healthy, are high in calories. A snack can easily add up to an extra 500 calories without your realizing it.

Be aware of the nutritional and caloric content of the foods you consume. As you can see, it's easy to hit 4,000 to 5,000 calories in a day. And it only takes 3,500 excess calories to create one new pound of fat on your body.

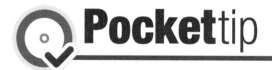

Pockettip

Nuts and nut butters are a great source of protein and healthy fats. Walnuts, pecans, cashews, Brazil nuts, pistachios and almonds are easy to package in plastic bags. Mix them with dry cereal for a healthy snack.

three

GOOD NUTRITION: YOU AND YOUR FOOD

Eating Healthy, Losing Weight

Your weight will ultimately be determined by calories consumed versus calories burned. A calorie is still a calorie, whether it is derived from fat, protein or carbohydrates. Calories are all equal in adding or decreasing body weight. All diets, including low-carb diets, can only be effective for long-term weight loss by limiting calories. The key to long-term weight loss is finding a convenient way to achieve a healthy balance of carbohydrates, protein and fat while maintaining an appropriate caloric intake.

Weight loss diets offer the reader many different approaches to manage the calories consumed. Some diets simply go too far with empty promises that take advantage of people's vulnerabilities.

If there is a "magic bullet" to controlling your weight it would be in your ability to control your portions and learning the caloric value of the foods you eat. How healthy you are is often a result of the nutritional content of the foods you choose to eat.

The Pocket Diet is a sustainable and healthy way to eat a variety of good food. When combined with an exercise regimen, it will help you achieve and maintain your desired weight and improve your overall health.

Remember, the most sustainable and safest way to lose weight is by reducing caloric intake to a level slightly lower than what your body burns through normal activity. Combine this with the consumption of well-balanced meals that include healthy food choices, and adopt a reasonable exercise regimen you can enjoy and sustain.

Start with a commitment to yourself to adopt and practice what you have learned in this book. Stay focused on that commitment, and the rewards of achieving a healthier weight and lifestyle will be inevitable. Your mind and body will need time to be redirected. You can achieve your goals if you are patient, forgiving and tenacious in your effort.

The New Food Pyramid

The U.S. Department of Agriculture (USDA) updated the U.S. Food Guide Pyramid in early 2005. When the old pyramid was developed in 1992, there was a lot less knowledge about and emphasis on whole grain foods than there is today. Also the link between exercise and staying healthy was not fully taken into consideration.

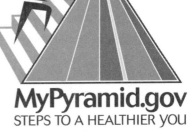

MyPyramid.gov
STEPS TO A HEALTHIER YOU

The new food pyramid is designed to provide a general guideline to healthy eating. Unlike the old pyramid, which showed only foods, it has been updated to include physical activity. The drawing of a person climbing stairs at the side of the new pyramid is a reminder that physical activity is as important to healthy living as eating well.

The bands are different widths to show how much of a particular food group a person should eat each day. So the orange band is wider than the yellow one because people need to eat more grains than fats and oils.

The pyramid also emphasizes the following points:

• Combine exercise with eating well. Food and exercise are closely linked. Exercise benefits every part of the body, including the mind. Experts now know that exercise fights off a range of possible health problems like heart disease, diabetes, and even depression. It is now recommended that people should strive to 60 minutes of moderate to vigorous exercise every day. This may be a challenge, but start small and try to work up to one hour over time.

- Eat a variety of foods. The different color bands in the pyramid send the message that it's important to eat lots of different foods. Not only does it provide people with a good balance of nutrients, but the variety of tastes helps develop an affinity for healthy foods.

Nutrition Facts: What They Are, How to Read Labels

Food labels—usually called Nutrition Facts—are valuable in making healthy eating an essential part of everyday meal planning. Most foods found in grocery stores today list their particular Nutrition Facts on a label typically located on the back or side of their package. Reading a food label is simple when you know what to look for.

Select your grocery items according to the following rules:

1. Is it a reasonable serving size? A good gauge is how many servings you could eat at one sitting.

2. Choose foods that are generally low in fat and high in fiber. Foods with less salt and less sugar, and those made with whole-grain ingredients are your best selections.

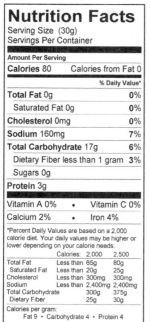

Serving Size

This is the most important piece of information on the label. It tells you how many servings are in the container. If one serving is one cookie, for example, and you eat three cookies, make sure you calculate the rest of the information on three servings (multiply by three).

Calories

How many calories are there per serving? Multiply the amount of calories by how many servings you actually had.

Sodium

Ready made processed foods are generally high in sodium. If you are on a sodium-restricted diet, choose foods that contain

140 milligrams or less of sodium per serving; aim for less than a total of 2,400 milligrams of sodium per day.

Fat
Not all fat is bad. In fact, fat is essential for hormone function and vitamin and mineral transport. Fat also makes food taste good! However, not all fats are healthy fats; saturated fat and trans-fats may contribute to heart disease. And fat has more than double the calories of protein and carbohydrates; therefore a smaller volume of high-fat foods contains more fat than a larger volume of low fat foods. So pay close attention to the fat content on food labels.

Carbohydrates, Sugar and Fiber
The total number of carbohydrates is reported on the nutrition facts panel along with the amount of sugar and fiber contained in one serving. Sugar is the simplest form of carbohydrate, and in the body all carbohydrate is broken down into sugar, or "glucose." Use the Nutrition Facts label to learn how many grams of sugar a product contains.

Also, when reviewing the ingredients in a food, look for foods that do not list sugar in the first three ingredients. Sugar may be listed under a number of names such as, brown sugar, dextrose, fructose, glucose, high fructose corn syrup, lactose, maltose, malt syrup, raw sugar, sucrose, and syrup. For example, when comparing breakfast cereals, choose the brand that contains the least amount of added sugar and most fiber. Fiber helps the human body with a number of tasks, including aiding in normal bowel function, promoting regularity, and controlling blood sugar levels. It also reduces risk of colon cancer and lowers blood cholesterol. To reach the recommended fiber intake of 25-35 grams per day, look for foods that contain at least 3 grams of fiber.

The Skinny on Fats

Fats occur naturally in food and are added to food products. They play an important role in nutrition by providing a concentrated source of energy for the body.

The body uses fat to store energy, insulate body tissue, and transport fat-soluble vitamins through the blood. Fats also enhance the flavor of food and make baked products tender. Some fat however may have negative effects on cholesterol and total health (see below to learn how to judge).

The Good, Not-So-Good, and Really Dangerous
Not all fats are created equal. There are four types:

1. Monounsaturated Fats (Good) are liquid at room temperature, but become solid when refrigerated. Examples of these fats include olive oil and canola oil. Monounsaturated fats may help improve cholesterol levels if used to replace saturated fats in the diet.

2. Polyunsaturated Fats (Good) remain liquid even while refrigerated. One type of polyunsaturated fat is worth special note: Omega - 3 fatty acids (Good) are special fats essential for normal body function, they are important components of cell membranes throughout the body, especially the eyes, brain and sperm cells. These fats regulate blood clotting, contraction and relaxation of the artery walls and inflammation. They have been shown to have significant benefits in the prevention of heart disease and stroke. The best sources of Omega-3s are fatty fish (like salmon), walnuts, flaxseed, and canola and soybean oil.

3. Saturated Fats (Bad) are solid at room temperature and include beef fat, butter, etc. These fats are typically found in animals and some plants and may increase bad cholesterol (LDL).

4. Trans-Fats (Bad) are artificially made through the hydrogenation of unsaturated fats. They are found in certain processed foods, may raise bad cholesterol (LDL) and lower good cholesterol (HDL).

The amount of fat eaten is as important as the types of fat consumed. Food fats consist of units called fatty acids that raise or lower blood cholesterol. Eat all types of fat in moderation, because fats contain more than twice the calories of proteins or carbohydrates.

The American Heart Association recommends keeping calories from fat at 25-35% of total calories consumed and saturated fats at less then 10% of total calories. For example, if you are consuming a diet of 1500 calories

Total Fat:

> 1500 calories x 30% = 450 calories from fat
> 450 calories from fat / 9 calories per gram = 50 grams of total fat per day

Saturated Fat:

> 1500 calories x 10% = 150 calories from saturated fat
> 150 calories from saturated fat / 9 calories per gram = 16 grams of saturated fat per day

The Danger of Trans-fats

Nevertheless, trans-fats should be avoided altogether. They are formed by the partial hydrogenation of vegetable oil, a chemical process that alters its nutrients. Hydrogenation solidifies oil to make it resemble real foods, such as butter. It is used to add texture to food products and to increase their shelf life.

Trans-fats have no nutritional value. In fact, studies show that trans-fats can be detrimental to your health. As a result, beginning in January 2006 the FDA required manufacturers to list all trans-fats on nutritional labels and some cities are now banning them from use in restaurants.

Daily Fat Intake Guide - 1 gram of fat = 9 calories				
Calorie Level	Total Fat Grams	Saturated Fat Grams	Reduced Fat Diet	
			Total Fat Grams	Saturated Fat Grams
1,500	45	15	33	10
1,800	55	18	40	13
2,000	60	20	45	14
2,200	66	22	50	16

Type of Fatty Acid	Effect on Cholesterol	Found In	Daily Usage
Monounsaturated	Lowers bad, Raises good	Avocados, peanuts, peanut oil, canola oil and olive oil.	10 to 15% of total calories
Polyunsaturated	Lowers bad	Vegetable oils (safflower, sunflower, corn), sunflower seeds. Main fats in seafood.	10% of total calories
Saturated	Raises bad	Animal fat, (butter, whole milk, ice cream, meat, poultry skin) coconut and palm oil.	Less than 10% of total calories
Trans	Raises bad, Lowers good	Hydrogenated vegetable fats (shortening, margarine), fried foods, baked goods, snacks.	Avoid

Cholesterol - The Good and the Bad

Every person's blood has cholesterol. Cholesterol helps produce cell membranes and hormones and serves other important functions. The body generates all of the cholesterol it needs; however, additional cholesterol may be derived from the consumption of meats, eggs, fish, poultry, cheese, milk and other animal products. In addition, some foods may trigger the body to produce extra cholesterol. These include products containing trans-fats and saturated fats.

If the cholesterol content of the blood stream gets too high, cholesterol particles begin sticking to the walls of the blood vessels and arteries, slowly narrowing the passageway and restricting blood flow. This condition is called arteriosclerosis, and a symptom of heart disease. Over 100 million American have total cholesterol of 200 mg/dl or higher and either have developed or are at risk for developing cardiovascular disease.

Maintaining normal cholesterol levels (less than 200 mg/dl) is a proven way to prevent cardiovascular disease. Eating foods low in saturated fat and cholesterol and avoiding trans-fats will help with this, as will physical exercise. Also, visit your doctor every 1-2 years, especially if you're over 40, to determine if your levels of total cholesterol, HDL and LDL, are in a safe range.

Good vs. Bad Cholesterol

In addition to maintaining an overall cholesterol level of 200 mg/dl or less, it is also important to know how much of your cholesterol is "good" and how much is "bad."

Cholesterol and other fats do not dissolve in blood and have to be transported to cells in your body with carriers called lipoproteins. There are two types of lipoproteins:

- High-Density Lipoproteins (HDL) which carry cholesterol away from the arteries and back to the liver where they are cleansed from the body. HDL is the "good" (or Healthy) cholesterol.

- Low-density lipoproteins (LDL) may deposit cholesterol and other substances on artery walls, causing the artery to narrow. LDL is the "bad" (or Lousy) cholesterol. Saturated fats and trans-fats contribute to increases in LDL levels.

You can raise your good (HDL) cholesterol by exercising, not smoking and staying at a healthy weight.

Proteins: The Body's Building Blocks

Protein and fat are the building materials of the body. Proteins are everywhere in the body – in our muscles, organs, tissue, bones, brain cells, blood cells, genetic matter, skin, hair and fingernails, etc.

Protein is essential for healthy living because it supports the constant repair and renewal that takes place inside our bodies.

Because the body cannot store protein, it must be replenished daily. The best protein sources are egg whites, legumes (beans), soy products, grains, poultry, fish and low-fat dairy products because they are low in fat and cholesterol.

The Important of Fiber

Many health experts advise people of all ages to consume more dietary fiber. There is considerable research suggesting that a diet with 25-35 grams of daily fiber may reduce the incidence of diabetes, heart disease, colon cancer and obesity.

Even though fiber is one of the most important components of a healthy diet, most Americans consume less than half the daily requirement. Fiber has no calories because the body cannot absorb it; however, it is essential for healthy bowel movements.

Insufficient dietary fiber is the usual cause of chronic constipation. This can lead to a myriad of other health problems such as hemorrhoids and varicose veins, which result from excessive straining when passing a stool. It is normal to have 1-2 easily passed bowel movements a day.

The American Dietetic Association recommends the following daily fiber consumption:

- Adults: 25-35 grams
- Children: Their age plus 5-10 grams each day

There are two types of dietary fiber: soluble and insoluble. Insoluble fiber passes through your digestive tract largely intact. It provides the bulk needed for proper stool formation. Insoluble fiber is found in most fruits, vegetables, whole-wheat breads, grains, wheat and corn bran, whole grains, and legumes. Adequate amounts of liquid are needed for this fiber to be effective.

Soluble fiber, which forms a gel when mixed with liquid, works in conjunction with insoluble fiber by helping to form the stool. Soluble fiber may also lower cholesterol by removing bile acids that digest saturated fat. Soluble fiber can also slow the absorption of sugars after a meal, thus reducing the amount of insulin the pancreas must produce. Stabilizing insulin levels reduces the stress on the pancreas. Soluble fiber is found in many fruits and vegetables, oat bran, oatmeal, barley and beans.

Simple Ways to Incorporate Fiber

- Add bran to muffins, pancake batter, casseroles, breakfast cereals, salads and yogurt.

- Boost the fiber content in cereals with fresh fruit and a sprinkling of bran.

- Choose whole-grain baked goods with raisins or other dried fruits.

Sodium: Good, but in Moderation

Salt contains sodium, an essential mineral for maintaining life. It controls our body's ability to retain water and maintains the critical balance between cells and body fluids. It also aids in the contraction of muscle tissue and serves as a vital ingredient in blood plasma and digestive secretions.

Excessive salt intake, however, may aggravate high blood pressure, hypertension and cardiovascular problems.

The National Academy of Sciences recommends that Americans consume a minimum of 500 mg of sodium per day to maintain normal body functions. Consuming up to 2,500 mg per day is still considered safe.

Unfortunately, the sodium intake of most Americans averages closer to 5,000-7,000 mg per day, most of it coming from processed and ready-made foods.

Ways to Reduce Salt Intake

- Cook from scratch. Reduce the consumption of prepared foods containing large amounts of sodium
- Instead of using salt, squeeze fresh lemon juice on steamed vegetables, broiled fish, rice or pasta for a refreshing taste
- Season your food with fresh herbs, wines, peppers and alternate spices, as well as with vegetable and citrus juice

- Choose fresh, frozen or canned vegetables that don't have added salt
- Snack on fresh fruits and vegetables, which are naturally low in sodium
- Enjoy salty snacks in moderation.

Carbohydrates: The Staff of Life

Carbohydrates have become a hot topic of debate ever since the introduction of the high-protein diet, which advocates a dramatic reduction in carbohydrate intake to reduce weight. However, carbohydrates help the body perform vital functions:

- They are the primary source of the body's energy
- They have a protein-sparing effect that protects muscle tissue from breaking down
- They are the primary fuel source for the brain
- They provide many important nutrients, including dietary fiber, which is essential for the digestive track

Carbohydrates can be complex or simple. Complex carbohydrates are good because they contain cellulose/fiber, are very important for digestion and may also help prevent colon cancer. Most Americans consume less than half of the recommended daily amount of dietary fiber, which should be approximately 30 grams per day.

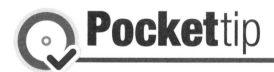
Pockettip

Make healthy food look smaller. The tricks the brain plays work both ways -- if making food look bigger helps us eat less, then making food look smaller helps us eat more. Serve your salad in a huge salad bowl, it won't seem like as much food. Put your vegetables on a big plate and your entree on a small one. You'll be satisfied with the entree and not overwhelmed by the salad.

four

FITNESS: A LIFETIME COMMITMENT

Introducing Exercise into Your Life

Nutrition and fitness experts agree that if you want to lose weight faster and keep it off you need to start and maintain an ongoing fitness program. This can be accomplished with only 30 minutes of activity per day. Every motion your body makes burns calories. The more you move, the more you lose!

Fitness Facts

• Even something as simple as a brisk, two-block walk every day can help you lose 10 pounds a year!

• Living healthfully is living happily. Exercise releases your brain's endorphins, powerful, naturally produced analgesics that make you feel better.

• Regular exercise is a great way to reduce stress. Research shows that headaches, chronic pain and other common physical conditions are aggravated by everyday stress. A 15-minute walk is a natural way to promote health–and, best of all, it's free.

One sure way to insure fitness success is to make it fun. Follows are some suggestions in finding an activity that will hopefully become a lifelong habit.

1. *Do what you like.* Because physical activity is only effective when you actually do it, choose something you enjoy. If running bores you, don't run. Go for a bike ride, try a new aerobics or boxing class. Keep trying new ways to get active until you find something you enjoy.

2. *Start slow.* If you are new to exercise or have not exercised in a while, begin slowly, such as with a walking program.

3. *Don't do it alone.* Exercise with a friend, family member or co-worker. A partner increases enjoyment, decreases boredom and helps to keep you motivated.

4. *Be flexible, but make it a priority.* Do what and when you can, but make sure exercise is a part of your schedule.

5. *Listen to music.* Music helps time pass quickly. It also will improve your endurance and tolerance for repetitive physical activity.

6. *Add variety to your fitness routine.* Choose more than one type of physical activity. This not only prevents boredom but works different muscle groups. Select an indoor and an outdoor activity to allow for changes in the weather or your schedule.

If you are uncertain what to do or where to start, you seek advice from a trainer or other fitness professional.

Walking is a Great Place to Start

One of the most convenient and low-risk ways to get started with a fitness program is by walking. A regular walking program can help reduce blood cholesterol, lower blood pressure, increase cardiovascular endurance, boost bone strength, burn calories, and keep weight down.

Walking Tips

1. Start out slowly. Going too far or too fast too soon is the number one cause of injuries. Start with a comfortable distance and then try to add five minutes each week until you reach 60 minutes.

2. Intermittent sessions are just as effective as continuous ones. If your health or schedule does not permit a 20- to 60-minute session of walking, break your sessions down into 10- to 15-minute intervals throughout the day.

3. Know your target heart rate. Most healthy individuals can exercise at between 60- 80% of their maxium heart rate. Find the zone where you are going to see the most benefit with the least amount of risk. The chart on Page 43 will help measure your resting heart rate.

4. Warm up for 5- 10 minutes by walking at a slow pace and gradually increasing speed until you reach your target heart rate. At the end of your session, walk slowly for 5- 10 minutes until your heart rate nears pre-exercise levels.

5. Stop walking if you experience pain, dizziness, severe shortness of breath, or any unusual signs or symptoms. If the condition persists, seek medical attention.

6. Drink water before, during, and after your walk. Take a bottle or container of water to avoid dehydration.

7. Add variety by alternating intervals of slow, moderate, and fast paces. You can also walk up hills, on trails, or increase the distance to continue progressing. Never walk while carrying wrist or ankle weights as they can cause unnecessary stress on your joints.

8. Prepare for your environment. That may mean dressing in layers that you can take off as you get warmer, or wearing synthetic fabrics to draw moisture from your skin. Always wear a hat and sunscreen.

9. Choose properly fitted footwear that is supportive and cushioned.

10. Be safe. Walk in a secure area or with a buddy. Carry a cell phone. If you wear a headset, keep the volume low so you can be aware of your surroundings.

What's your Heart Rate?

Exercise and a good fitness program can play an important part of overall weight loss and fat reduction. Target Heart Rate, or THR, is a common way of judging how hard you should exercise during endurance activities. It tells you how fast the average person should try to make his or her heart beat during endurance sessions. While exercising it is essential that the exercise being undertaken is done correctly, not just to avoid injury but also to ensure that maximum results are achieved in the shortest time possible.

If an individual is exercising too hard their heart rate will be outside the ideal heart rate zone and they will be at risk of injury or burn out. It is unnecessary to be working at this rate and will not result in weight loss or overall fitness occurring more quickly. Easing off a little will result in the heart rate being in the correct zone and be the most affective.

Heart rate at the lower end of the zone means that an individual is not working hard enough, and as a result the heart rate will be below the ideal zone. The further from the ideal zone the more ineffective the exercise will be. Exercise in this range may end in frustration in the long term as the desired increases in fitness and reduction in weight and body fat will not be seen.

Heart rate should be monitored regularly throughout exercise to ensure that the rate is in the ideal range.

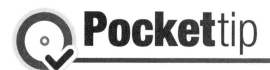

Pockettip

Don't overdo it. Do low- to-moderate-level activities, especially at first. You can slowly increase their duration and intensity as you become more fit. Over time, work up to exercising on most days of the week for 30-60 minutes.

Measuring Your Target Heart Rate

How to take your pulse: Place your index and middle finger around the back side of your wrist (approximately one inch down from the top of your wrist on the thumb side). Find your pulse and count for six seconds. Multiply this number by 10. Try to keep this number in your target zone.

Age in Years	Average Maximum Heart Rate	Target Heart Rate for Exercise at 60-80% of Maximum Heart Rate
20	200	120-160
30	190	114-152
40	180	108-144
50	170	102-136
60	160	96-128
70	150	90-120

Stretching, Aerobics, and Strength Training
Keeping It Balanced

A balanced fitness program consists of three components: stretching, aerobics and strength training.

Stretching

Regular stretching can help reduce pain, improve muscle imbalances, and decrease your chance of injury.

Stretching Tips

1. Stretch after exercise, when your muscles are warm and more receptive to deeper stretching

2. Focus on the muscle you are stretching and keep all the other muscles relaxed

3. Move into each stretch slowly, until you feel mild tension in the muscle and never bounce

4. If you feel pain, you've stretched too far

5. Breathe deeply, slowly and rhythmically while holding the stretch and never hold your breath

6. Hold each stretch for at least 10-30 seconds, then release

7. A stretch can be repeated several times before moving on to another stretch

8. After you have held a stretch, relax that muscle group and try to stretch again, going a little further each time

9. Ideally, you should spend at least 30 minutes three times a week, on flexibility training

10. The practice of yoga or Pilates will also help enhance flexibility.

Stretch Program

Finger stretching – to maintain finger dexterity. With the palm of the right hand facing down, gently force your fingers back toward your forearm. Use the left hand for leverage, then place the left hand on top of your other hand and push your fingers down. Suggested repetitions: Five on each hand.

Hand rotation – to maintain wrist flexibility and range of motion. Grasp your right wrist with your left hand. Keep your right palm facing down. Slowly rotate your hand five times each way, clockwise, then counter-clockwise. Suggested repetitions: Five on each hand.

Ankle and foot circling – to improve flexibility and range of motion of ankles. Cross your right leg over the opposite knee, rotating your foot slowly, making large complete circles. Suggested repetitions: 10 rotations to the right, 10 to the left on each leg.

Neck extension– to improve flexibility and range of motion of neck. Sit up comfortably. Bend your head forward until your chin touches your chest. You may want to stretch forward by simply jutting your chin out. Return to starting position and slowly rotate your head to the left. Then return to starting position and slowly rotate your head to the right. Suggested repetitions: 5.

Single knee pull – to stretch the lower back and back of the leg. Lie on your back, hands at your sides. Pull one leg up to your chest, grasp with both arms and hold for five counts. Repeat with the opposite leg. Suggested repetitions: 3 - 5.

Simulated crawl stroke/back stroke/breast stroke – to stretch shoulders. Stand with your feet shoulder-width apart, arms at your sides, in a relaxed position. Bend your knees and alternately swing right and left arms backwards, upward, and forward as if swimming. Suggested repetitions: 6 - 8 movements on each stroke.

Reach– to stretch shoulders and rib cage. Take a deep breath, extending your arms overhead. If standing, rise on your toes while reaching. Exhale slowly, lowering your arms. This exercise can be done in a seated position. Suggested repetitions: 6 - 8.

Backstretch– to improve the flexibility of the lower back. Sit up straight, bend far forward and straighten up. Repeat, clasping your hands on your left knee. Repeat by clasping your hands on your right knee. Exhale while bending forward. Suggested repetitions: 4 - 6 over each knee.

Chain breaker– to stretch chest muscles. Stand erect, with your feet about six inches apart. Tighten your leg muscles, then draw your stomach in, hips forward. Extend chest, bringing your arms up with clenched fists. Take a deep breath, then exhale slowly. Slowly pull your arms back as far as possible, keeping your elbows at the same height as your chest. Suggested repetitions: 8 - 10.

Aerobics

Aerobic exercise not only helps you burn calories and lose weight more quickly, but research also shows that those who maintain a long-term aerobic program are more likely to keep the weight off.

There are several cardiovascular (aerobic) exercises to choose from and include jogging, brisk walking, swimming, biking, skiing and aerobic dancing, among others.

All aerobic exercise increases your heart rate and breathing. It makes no difference what form of exercise you choose as long as you get your heart rate up. So the best exercise for you is the exercise that you enjoy and do on a regular basis.

The Importance of Strength Training

Most of us know that exercise is an important component to getting healthy and losing body fat, but we tend to equate it with aerobic activity like jogging, walking or cycling. We often forget that strength training offers just as many health benefits as aerobic exercise. You can expect to experience the following benefits after initiating a strength training program.

- Improved posture
- Increased bone density
- Reduced risk for injury
- Increased muscular strength and endurance
- Improved muscle tone
- Increased fat loss
- Increased metabolic rate

Muscle comprises approximately 40% of our total body weight. By developing your muscular system, you will significantly increase your metabolism. Muscle is an energy burning tissue and the more of it that you have in your body, the more fat you will burn both during exercise and during rest. In fact, one pound of muscle tissue expends an additional 30-40 calories per day. That may not sound like a lot but consider that after an 8-12 week strength training program you can expect to develop 2-4 lbs of lean muscle tissue. That equates to an extra 90 to 160 calories being burned a day. Multiply that by 365 days per year and we're talking about 10-14 lbs of fat either lost or not gained compared to not having that lean muscle mass. Now that's motivation to get strength training!

Strength training can transform your body into a desirable shape and help defy the aging process. It does not need to be time-consuming or expensive to produce health and fitness benefits. The goal is to develop and maintain a significant amount of muscle mass to increase metabolism.

Strength Training Program

Arm curl– to strengthen arm muscles. Use a weighted object such as a book, a can of vegetables or small dumbbell. Stand or sit erect with arms at your sides, holding the weighted object. Bend your arm, raising the weight, then lower it. This can be done while seated. Suggested repetitions: 10-15 each arm.

Arm extension – to tone muscles in the back of the arm. Sit or stand erect with your arms at their sides. Lift a weighted object of less than five pounds overhead. Slowly bend your arm until you reach the back of your head Suggested repetitions: 10-15 each arm.

Modified knee push-up – to strengthen upper back, chest, and back of arms. Start on bent knees, with your hands on the floor, moving slightly forward with your shoulders. Lower your body until your chin touches the floor. Return to starting position. Suggested repetitions: 5-10.

Calf raise – to strengthen lower legs and ankles. Stand erect with your hands on hips or on the back of a chair for balance. Spread your feet apart 6-12 inches. Slowly raise your body to your toes, lifting your heels. Return to starting position. Suggested repetitions: 10-15.

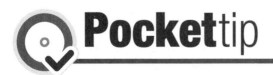

Pockettip

Keep a record of your activities. Reward yourself at special milestones. Nothing motivates like success!

Alternate leg lunges – to strengthen upper thighs and inside legs and to stretch back of legs. Take a comfortable stance with your hands on your hips. Step forward 18-24 inches with your right leg. Keep your left heel on the floor. Push off with your right leg and resume standing position. Suggested repetitions: 5-10 each leg.

Modified sit-up – to improve abdominal strength. Lie on your back, feet on the floor with your finger tips behind your ears. Look straight up at the ceiling and lift your head and shoulders off floor. Suggested repetitions: 10.

Side lying leg lift – to strengthen and tone outside of thigh and hip muscles. Lie on your right side, legs extended. Raise both legs 4-5 inches. Lower to starting position. Suggested repetitions: 10 on each side.

Physical Activity and Calories Burned

Medical and fitness experts measure physical exertion as a MET value (Metabolic equivalent). This is a multiple of oxygen consumption during rest. 1 MET equals 3.5ml/kg/min., which is the amount of oxygen that a person needs while at rest. For example, 13 METs as a result of an exercise test means the person can exceed his resting oxygen consumption 13 times.

To determine the calories you are expending per hour, multiply your weight in kilograms by the MET value given in the chart below. To find your body weight in kilograms, divide your weight in pounds by 2.2. For example, 150 pounds divided by 2.2 equals 68 kilograms. Multiply this figure by the MET value to determine how many calories you will burn per hour while engaged in that activity. A 150-pound person engaged in an hour of high-impact aerobics would expend 477 calories.

MET Value	Physical Activity
6.0	Aerobic Dance, general
7.0	Aerobic Dance, high-impact
5.0	Aerobic Dance, low-impact
7.0	Backpacking
5.5	Ballroom Dancing, fast
3.0	Ballroom Dancing, slow
8.0	Basketball game
4.0	Bicycling > 10 miles per hour, leisure ride
6.0	Bicycling 10-12 miles per hour, slow
8.0	Bicycling 12-14 miles per hour, moderate
10.0	Bicycling 14-16 miles per hour, vigorous
12.0	Bicycling 16-19 miles per hour, racing
16.0	Bicycling > 20 miles per hour, racing
5.0	Bicycling Stationary, light effort
7.0	Bicycling Stationary, moderate effort
12.5	Bicycling Stationary, very vigorous effort
10.5	Bicycling Stationary, vigorous effort
3.0	Bowling
8.0	Calisthenics, heavy effort
4.5	Calisthenics, light or moderate effort, (e.g., push-ups, pull-ups, sit-ups)
8.0	Circuit Training, general
6.0	Elliptical Training, general
5.5	Golf, carrying clubs
4.5	Golf, general
6.5	Horseback Riding, trotting
3.5	House Cleaning, general
7.0	Jogging, general
10.0	Jumping Rope, moderate
10.0	Karate, Kickboxing, Tae Kwan Do, Judo
8.5	Mountain Biking
5.5	Mowing Lawn, general, push mower
7.0	Racquetball, casual
8.0	Rock or Mountain Climbing

MET Value	Physical Activity
7.0	Roller Skating
9.5	Rowing Stationary, general
3.5	Rowing Stationary, light effort
7.0	Rowing Stationary, moderate effort
12.0	Rowing Stationary, very vigorous effort
8.5	Rowing Stationary, vigorous effort
8.0	Running > 5 miles per hour
10.0	Running > 6 miles per hour
11.5	Running > 7 miles per hour
13.5	Running > 8 miles per hour
15.0	Running > 9 miles per hour
9.5	Ski Machine, general
7.0	Skiing, general
8.0	Stair Climbing, general
8.0	Swimming Laps, moderate effort
4.0	Tai Chi
7.0	Tennis, general
3.0	Volleyball, general
3.0	Walking > 3 miles per hour
4.0	Walking > 3.5 miles per hour
4.0	Water Aerobics
6.0	Weight Lifting, machine or free weight, vigorous
4.0	Yoga, Hatha

five

THE POCKET DIET MEAL PLAN

How Many Calories Do You Need?

Achieving your ideal weight begins with finding the right balance of exercise and caloric intake. Each person's balance is unique. The best way to find out your personal caloric needs is to have your metabolism tested. Metabolism testing measures the amount of oxygen burned while resting. Testing also calculates how many calories you would burn in a day if you rested the entire day. This test can help you determine how many calories you should be eating each day to maintain, gain or lose weight. To have your metabolism tested locally visit www.korr.com.

You can choose from three meal plans on the Pocket Diet. These depend on your size, *activity level and personal goals.* Meal plans are designed to provide you with the appropriate amounts of carbohydrates, protein, and fat to achieve a weight loss of 1-2 pounds per week.

The Pocket Diet allows you to eat a variety of healthy, tasty foods. However, you must pay close attention to both portion sizes and amount of food you eat.

Meals and the Pocket Diet

The most frequently asked question about the Pocket Diet is: "Do I really have to eat all my meals in a pita pocket?"

It's not necessary all the time, but if you want a simple and effective way to control portions while developing healthy eating habits, pocket bread is the key. This is what the study group discovered. It is also a critical and convenient source of complex carbohydrates and perfect for breakfast, lunch and some dinner meals.

Portion control is the essence of any successful diet, including the Pocket Diet. You can't overfill a pocket like a sandwich or your plate. We believe that you will find, as did the 38 members in the Community Memorial Hospital study, that the Kangaroo pocket is a convenient, healthy and delicious way to eat your favorite foods and control your portions. However, for meals without bread, or when you want a change, just select another complex carb equivalent to the pocket bread from the "Pocket Bread Equivalent Chart" in the appendix section on page 246.

About the Kangaroo Pocket

Kangaroo Pocket bread is a fat-free, wholesome bread made with unbleached white, whole wheat, or whole grain flour. It has a delicious light, hearth- baked flavor that compliments the taste of all foods. The exact nutritional content varies by variety, but a 1.3-ounce whole wheat pocket contains approximately 80 calories and 16 grams of carbohydrates, with 4 grams of fiber, and 3 grams of protein. By comparison, two slices of traditional sandwich bread, bagels, buns or muffins have significantly more calories and carbs than a Kangaroo Pocket.

Substituting a Kangaroo Pocket for traditional sliced bread, bagels or buns can lead to a significant reduction in calories every week.

Basic Meal Plans

The following sample meal plans on page (53) are based on the average number of calories in the pita pocket recipes. Plan-A has 1400 calories; Plan-B, 1800 calories; and Plan-C, 2200 calories.

To determine the meal plan that best fits your body type and activity level, use the following guidelines with a calorie range for the body types described next page. To obtain your exact caloric requirement and select the appropriate Pocket Diet meal plan, you may want to consult a registered dietitian or visit: www.korr.com.

Increasing physical activity is a key factor in the success of the Pocket Diet. When you first begin the Pocket Diet, you might want to select the Pocket Meals that are below the average calorie recipe.

As you boost your physical activity, you can incorporate some higher calorie recipes within the same plan.

Select Meal Plan A (1,200 to 1,600 calories a day) if you are:
- a small woman who exercises regularly
- a small or medium woman who wants to lose weight
- a medium woman who does not exercise much

Select Meal Plan B (1,600 to 2,000 calories a day) if you are:
- a medium woman who exercises regularly
- a large woman who wants to lose weight
- a small man at a healthy weight
- a medium man who does not exercise much
- a medium to large man who wants to lose weight

Select Meal Plan C (2,000 to 2,400 calories a day) if you are:
- a medium to large man who exercises regularly, or has a physically active job
- a large man at a healthy weight
- a large woman who exercises regularly, or has a physically active job

	Plan A 1200 - 1600	Plan B 1600 - 2000	Plan C 2000-2400
A small woman who exercises regularly	■		
A small woman who wants to lose weight	■		
A medium woman who does not exercise much	■		
A medium woman who exercises regularly		■	
A large woman who wants to lose weight		■	
A small man at a healthy weight who exercises regularly		■	
A medium man who does exercise		■	
A medium to large man who wants to lose weight		■	
A medium to large man who exercises regularly, or has a physically active job			■
A large man at a healthy weight			■
A large woman who exercise regularly or has a physically active job			■

Adapted from: National Institute of Health (www.niddk.nih.gov)

Three Meal Plans

Eating a variety of the recipes during the week is important for well-balanced nutrition, and to ensure that not just the higher calorie meals are being consumed.

For beverages, choose water most often. However, 4-8 ounces of 100% fruit juice, skim or lowfat milk, or sugar free soda and tea may be consumed at each meal.

Plan A
Average of 1,400 calories/day

Breakfast	1 Pita Pocket Meal with skim milk	or	1 cup whole grain cereal
Snack:	Snack from list		
Lunch	1 Pita Pocket Meal	with	1 cup raw veggies
Snack	1 Pita Pocket Meal	or	Snack from list
Dinner	2 Pita Pocket Meals with 1/2 cup veggies 1 cup vegetables or dressing)	or	3 oz lean protein 3/4 cup whole grain starch 2 tsp fat (olive oil, butter
Snack:	Snack from List		

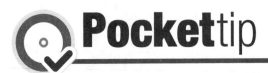

Pockettip

Incorporate quick and easy meals into your meal planning process. If your family loves sloppy Joes – cook up the sloppy joe meat in bulk and freeze it – then all you need to do is defrost the meat, grab some pocket and viola.

Plan B
Average of 1,800 calories/day

Breakfast	1 Pita Pocket Meal with skim milk	or	1.5 cup whole grain cereal
Snack	1 Pita Pocket Meal	or	Snack from list
Lunch	2 Pita Pocket Meals	with	1 cup raw veggies
Snack	1 Pita Pocket Meal	or	Snack from list
Dinner	2 Pita Pocket Meals With 1/2 cup veggies 1 cup vegetables or dressing)	or	5 oz lean protein 1 cup whole grain starch 2 tsp fat (olive oil, butter
Snack:	Snack from list		

Plan C
Average of 2,200 calories/day

Breakfast	2 Pita Pocket Meals with skim milk	or	2 cup whole grain cereal
Snack	2 Pita Pocket Meals	or	Snack from list
Lunch	2 Pita Pocket Meals	with	1 cup raw veggies
Snack	2 Pita Pocket Meal	or	Snack from list
Dinner	2 Pita Pocket Meals With 1/2 cup veggies 1 cup vegetables or dressing)	or	6 oz lean protein 1 cup whole grain starch 1 Tbs fat (olive oil, butter
Snack:	Snack from list		

Sample Meal Plan - Food Selections

Meal Plan: Breakfast	A – 1,400	B – 1,800	C – 2,200
Recipe : walnut Spread	1-Veggie scramble	1-Date Tomato	2-Bacon Cheese
Pocket Bread	1-Pocket bread	1-Pocket bread	2-Pocket bread
AM Snack : 1/2 cup low fat : cottage cheese **Lunch**	1 small banana	1 orange 1/2 cup low fat cottage cheese	1 grapefruit
Recipe	1-Chicken salad	2-Tuna salad	2-Shrimp salad
Pocket Bread	1-Pocket bread & baked potato chips	2-Pocket bread	2-Pocket bread
Vegetable	1 cup raw veggies	1 cup raw veggies	1 cup raw veggies
PM Snack : 1 apple :	1/4 cup almonds and seeds 1 banana	1/2 cup yogurt	1/2 cup mixed nuts
Dinner			
Recipe	2-Philly cheese steak	2-Chicken stir fry	2-Garbanzo chicken
Pocket Bread	2-Pocket bread	2-Pocket bread	2-Pocket bread
Vegetable : (in stir fry)	1/2 cup veggies	1/2 cup veggies	1 cup veggies
PM Snack	3 graham crackers	1/4 cup nuts	1/2 cup sherbet

Eat foods in moderation. Not all foods within a category are created equal. For example, whole, fresh apples should be consumed more often than apple pie, and a person should try to get most of their dairy intake from low-fat milk instead of cream cheese or other high-fat dairy products

Some tips on making selections include:
- Make half your grains whole grains
- Vary your veggies
- Focus on fruit
- Consume calcium rich foods (low fat dairy products, enriched soy products, green leafy vegetables, etc.)
- Go lean with protein (turkey and chicken breasts, beef and pork tenderloins) egg whites, tofu, fish, etc.).

Out of Pocket Meals

Once you learn how to control your potion size by using the about of food that fits into a pita pocket, you can start introducing other (non-pita) meals into your diet. We call these "Out of Pocket" meals

Be sure to try to eat breakfast every day. It will help you control your hunger later in the day.

How to Pick a Breakfast Cereal

The healthiest breakfast is whole grain cereal. If you're trying to lose weight, control cholesterol or diabetes, or just need a lot of energy, one great option is a hot cooked cereal of whole grains, such as oatmeal; or barley, brown rice or wheat berries cooked and served like oatmeal - perhaps with cinnamon or raisins.

If you prefer cold cereal, you need to check the list of ingredients carefully. The FIRST ingredient should be a whole grain. Then scan through the entire list and if you see the words "partially hydrogenated," put the box back on the shelf. You should avoid foods with partially hydrogenated oils (or "trans fats"), and they show up in an alarming number of cereal brands (see the list below.)

Once you've eliminated all the brands made with refined grains or partially hydrogenated oils, check for added sugars (you want little or none) and fiber (you want a lot.)

The fiber content listed on the nutrition label can be confusing because it's based on serving size, and very light cereals (such as puffed wheat) show little fiber per serving, but an acceptable amount when you adjust for weight. Cereals made from bran (the outer covering removed from whole grains) will have higher fiber content than cereals made from whole grains (which have the germ and starchy parts of the grains as well as the fiber), but they can be hard to digest.

Recommended: Cereals made from Whole Grains
(no trans fats, little or no added sugars when checked; but check the labels -- ingredients can change.)

Cheerios - General Mills
Chex, Wheat - General Mills
Grape Nuts - Post
Healthy Choice Toasted Brown Sugar Squares - Kelloggs
Kashi - Kashi Company
Mini-Wheats, Raisin Squares - Kelloggs
Mini-Wheats, Frosted, Bite-Size - Kelloggs
Mini-Wheats, Frosted - Kelloggs
Muesli - Familia
Nutri-Grain, Golden Wheat - Kelloggs
Nutri-Grain, Almond-Raisin - Kelloggs
Oatmeal Crisp, Almond - General Mills
Oatmeal Crisp, Apple Cinnamon - General Mills
Oatmeal Crisp, Raisin - General Mills
Oatmeal Squares - Quaker
Organic Healthy Fiber Multigrain Flakes - Health Valley
Puffed Wheat - Quaker
Shredded Wheat - Post
Shredded Wheat & Bran - Post
Shredded Wheat, Frosted - Post
Shredded Wheat, Spoon Size - Post
Uncle Sam - U.S. Mills
Wheaties, Crispy 'n' Raisins - General Mills

Recommended: All Bran or High Bran Cereals
(no trans fats, little or no added sugars.)

100% Bran - Post
All Bran, bran buds - Kelloggs
All-Bran, extra fiber - Kelloggs
All-Bran, original - Kelloggs
Bran Flakes - Post
Chex, Multi-Bran - General Mills
Complete Wheat Bran Flakes - Kelloggs
Complete Oat Bran Flakes - Kelloggs
Fiber 7 Flakes - Health Valley
Fiber One - General Mills
Oat Bran - Quaker
Oat Bran Flakes - Health Valley
Oat Bran Flakes with Raisins - Health Valley
Organic Bran with Raisins - Health Valley
Raisin Bran - Kelloggs
Raisin Bran Flakes - Health Valley
Raisin Bran, Whole Grain Wheat - Post
Total, Raisin Bran - General Mills

Out-of-Pocket Breakfast Recommendations
- ¾ – 1 cup cold cereal (from the approved list above)
  (select those cereals that are high-fiber, low-fat & low sugar)
- ½ cup skim milk
- ½ - ¾ fruit (fresh or frozen

The Pocket Plate

Every skill takes practice to perfect and portion control is no different. Now that you have perfected "in the pocket" portion control you may be wondering-- what do I do if I want to eat a meal without a pita pocket? The answer is simple, if you have been following the number of pita pockets recommended for your body type in The Pocket Diet you have already become used to the perfect portion size for your body. But, to make sure old habits (eating whatever portion is served) do not return we have a great tool for you:

- When grocery shopping purchase the plastic dinner plates that are divided into 3 sections

- Fill the largest section with non-starchy vegetables (listed on page 245

- Fill one of the small sections with Heart Healthy Proteins (listed on page 245

- Fill the final section with carbohydrates (use the Pita Bread Equivalent Guide on page 246

If you are dining out or do not have your sectioned plates available you can still use the same idea. Just divide your plate in half and fill one half with veggies. Split the other half with your protein and carbohydrates.

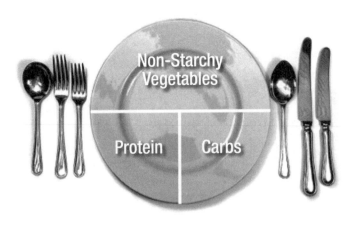

Still Hungry?

If you are still hungry after meals and between snacks while following your meal plan, increase your vegetables. Vegetables are full of water and high in fiber. Although they fill you up, they are low in calories. Try some of the veggies below:

Cucumbers	Broccoli
Asparagus	Spinach
Kale	Tomato
Celery	Carrots
Peppers	Sugar snap peas
Brussels sprouts	Cauliflower
Cabbage	Lettuce

Managing Snacks

The best way to ensure that you are eating the healthiest snacks is to have them readily available. Following are some tips for healthy snacking:

- Stock your pantry at home and your drawers at work.
- Eat a wide variety of these snacks.
- Eat something every 3-4 hours, and never wait until you are so hungry that you will eat anything.
- Also make sure you watch your portions.
- Eat the snacks one hour before your main meals to suppress your appetite.

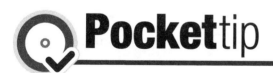

Pockettip

Use timesavers. Buy pre-cut and bagged lettuce for salad, baby carrots for stew, pre-cut fruit for a snack of use frozen vegetables.

Best Snack List

Snack Foods	Serving Size Average Calories	Serving Tips & Comments
Fresh Fruits Apple, orange, tangerine, pear, Kiwi, banana, cantaloupe, honey dew, plums, All berries, nectarine, mango, apricots, grapes (17 per serving)	1 med. size fruit /or 1/2 cup = 80 calories	Eat a variety of all these healthy fruits 2-3 per day
Veggies baby carrots, celery sticks, pickles, cauliflower, broccoli, cucumbers kohlrabi, fresh string beans, bell peppers… any fresh, non-starchy veggies you like!	1 cup = 80 calories	These are the most nutritious low calorie snacks you can eat. Dip them in a no fat low calorie dressing if you desire.
Nuts almonds, walnuts, unsalted roasted peanuts, sunflower seeds, toasted soy beans	1/4 cup, or approx. 15 nuts = 75 calorie	Tip: Buy these nuts in large 24 oz. bags and mix them all together in equal portions. Add some raisins for a bit of sweetness and fiber.
Pop Corn (easy salt no butter)	3 cups = 90 calories	
Dried fruit Apricots, figs, date, raisins	1/4 cup, or 4-5 pieces = 60 calories	These are hi- fiber, but high in natural sugar.
Yogurt Choose no fat low sugar variety	1/2 cup = 80 calories or 110 with a little fruit	Mix in fresh cut fruit: berries, pear, nectarine, peach
Cottage Cheese Choose no fat, or 2% fat	1/2 cup = 80-100 calories	Mix in low sugar fruit cocktail, or fresh cut peaches, nectarine
Frozen yogurt Fat Free, or Regular	1/3 cup = 80 calories	Try 1/4 cup, it maybe just enough to satisfy that sweet tooth after dinner
Sorbet / Sherbet	1/3 cup = 80 calories	

Planning Your Meals

As you familiarize yourself with the meal plans, please keep the following in mind:

1. A serving/portion size for the majority of recipes is approximately 3 ounces by weight, or 1/3 of a cup by volume, which equals the contents that a 6" Kangaroo Pocket can hold. If the portion serving size is less or more than that amount, it will be specified in the nutritional information in a recipe.

2. The recipe calories-per-serving listed in each meal plan are based on the average calories-per-serving for all the recipes in each meal section. Each recipe varies in caloric content. It assumes you are eating a variety of the recipes, which is recommended. We used an average of 85 calories for one Kangaroo Pocket which is not included in the calorie total for the recipe.

3. You can adjust the meal plans to a certain calorie level for your specific body and desired weight loss. The food quantity lists in this chapter should help with this.

4. Drink plenty of water. You can also have limited amounts of nonfat or lowfat (1%) milk and natural fruit juices (100% juice), but be sure and check the serving size, and incorporate the calorie count into your overall daily total. Diet soft drinks, ice tea, hot tea, coffee, or any others that contains no sugar are allowed. Avoid beverages with empty calories such as sweetened tea and colas.

5. Choose healthy snack foods from the "Best Snack List" on page 58.

6. You may substitute other complex carbs for the pocket bread. Check the pocket bread equivalent chart in the appendix on page 246.

7. Focus on eating the correct portions for each meal plan.

8. You do not have to eat all the food for each meal in one sitting. Grazing throughout the day is acceptable. Just keep track of what you eat.

9. Eating all types of foods is important for well-balanced nutrition, and for your enjoyment.

Make sure you eat a variety of the recipes during the week. Remember to eat slowly and savor your food. It takes your body 15-20 minutes to feel satisfied after you start eating.

Tips for Pocket Diet Success:

- Plan your weekly meals (very important).
- Stock your pantry with the foods on the plan. Get rid of unhealthy convenience food.
- Prepare enough food so that you will have leftovers for the next day.
- Do not worry if you overeat on any given day, just get back on track the next day. Missing one day will not have a significant impact on your diet.
- Focus on maintaining a daily / weekly average of your calorie goal.
- Stay within the total calories allowed for each

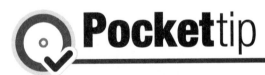

Pockettip

Before shopping, make a list by deciding which meals you're going to make during the coming week and include the ingredients on your shopping list. Don't forget to plan for breakfast and snacks, too. With a list at hand, you're less likely to stray from your diet to the tempting but unhealthy foods. As a bonus, you may also save time and money on grocery shopping by using a list.

Pocket Diet Recipes

About the Ingredients

The Pocket Diet is not about calorie counting, but about relearning portion control and learning to make the healthiest choices available. It's not a "No No" diet. You know, no carb, no fat, no flavor, no fun. This is an easily adaptable, go anywhere plan.

Low Fat: When choosing what to fill your pockets with, it's up to you what goes into them. In our recipes we recommend light and low fat ingredients whenever possible. This way you never feel the reduced calories, and your heart is healthier for it.

Vegetarian products are another healthy option, especially for kids. If your kids insist on chicken nuggets, try the vegetarian version (Quorn is great). Many come frozen or refrigerated and only need a quick zap in the microwave to complete your meal. Veggie Bacon is also a good option when you only need a slice or two and don't want to mess with cooking.

Pre-prepped vegetables can make your life easier, and healthier too. If buying peppers chopped, mushrooms sliced, and spinach washed means you'll actually use them, then the payoff is worth the price.

Pitas are available just about everywhere. Because they lack the preservative found in so many breads on the store shelves it's best to freeze them and thaw as you need. Whole-wheat pitas are a good choice for fiber and extra vitamins.

Frozen foods can keep you on track. Fresh isn't always available, and frozen cuts down on the number of times you need to shop for ingredients. So much is available frozen to help you eat healthier – grilled chicken strips, cooked shrimp, fruit, and a multitude of vegetables. Convenience foods can also keep you on track. Small frozen meals fit in a pita (Health Choice The Truth About Carbs, Michelina's) and are easier than take-out. Frozen vegetables and meats cut down on prep time, but still allow for sensible meals.

About Utensils: Equipping your Kitchen for The Pocket Diet

The entire focus of The Pocket Diet, and The Pocket Diet Cookbook is ease. We know you have too much to do, and not enough time to do it in as it is. That's why we've designed recipes that are easy to prepare, using as few ingredients and as little equipment as possible. We think you'll find most, of not all, of these tools in your kitchen already!

Baking Sheet – A flat cookie sheet or a sided jellyroll pan both work nicely.

Blender (hand or stand) – A must for making smoothies and slushes.

Box grater – cuts cheese and vegetables down to size.

Chef's knife – the heavy wide blade is a wonderful multipurpose tool.

Cutting boards – We recommend at least two of these, one for meats and one for vegetables. Use different colored boards to help you keep them separate. Always wash with soap and water before storing.

Food Processor – Chop, grate, slice, blend, and puree. This tool is a real timesaver in the kitchen.

Loaf pan – nice for standing up pitas while you warm them in the oven (metal) or microwave (glass).

Measuring cups & spoons – stainless steel or dollar store plastic.

Microwave Omelet pan – nothing makes omelets easier, and the convenient size is perfect for stuffing into a pita.

Nonstick skillet – a small (8 inch) is perfect for most needs, but a larger (14 inch) is nice when cooking for a crowd.

Rubber Spatula – Great for scraping bowls clean. If you have the silicone variety you can even use them to stir while you cook. Fewer dishes all around.

Stove-top Grill Pan – Round or griddle sized, these are wonderful for grilling vegetables, meats, and kabobs. Alternatively, a George Foreman grill can cut your cooking time almost in half.

Tongs – for turning meat and vegetables while grilling.

Vegetable peeler – removes skin from hard vegetables. Remember to always peel away from your body.

Wok – all the stir-fries included here can be made in a large nonstick skillet, but a wok is a great tool to have.

Not to mention these utensil drawer basics:

Can opener	Foil
Spatula	Wooden skewers

Pocket Diet Shopping List

Keep these ingredients on hand and you'll be able to make over half the recipes in this cookbook. Stock up on these basics and you'll be able to bypass the grocery store before dinner – the greatest time saver of all!

PRODUCE
Apples
Cabbage
Cucumber
Lettuce
Onions
Peppers
Sliced mushrooms
Sprouts
Strawberries
Tomatoes
Zucchini

BREADS
Kangaroo pita salad pockets whole wheat or whole grain

CANNED
Beans (garbanzo, kidney, black)
Fat free flavored refried beans
Mandarin oranges

Pineapple
Tomato paste

DAIRY

Blue cheese
Fat free ricotta
Light cream cheese
Light sour cream
Light yogurt (plain, vanilla)
Parmesan
Provolone
Reduced fat cheeses *(cheddar, mozzarella, Swiss, Monterey Jack)*

PROTEINS

Beef: ground sirloin, preformed burger patties, steak
Canned tuna (water packed)
Chicken breast, boneless skinless
Eggs, or egg substitute
Ground turkey
Hot dogs (turkey, or low fat beef)
Lunchmeat: roast beef, smoked turkey, roast turkey, turkey ham
Shrimp – cooked salad shrimp, cocktail shrimp
Turkey Bacon

FROZEN

Beef strips (Steak Ums)
Broccoli
Chicken nuggets
Corn
Fish Sticks
Grilled chicken strips
Spinach
Veggie Bacon
Veggie burger patties
Veggie Sausage

OILS/FATS

Cooking Spray – look for flavored sprays like butter, garlic, and olive oil
Olive Oil

CONDIMENTS

Balsamic vinegar
BBQ sauce
Bottled minced garlic
Dijon mustard
Light mayonnaise
Light ranch dressing
Peanut butter
Reduced fat pesto
Salsa
Sugar free preserves
Teriyaki sauce
Worcestershire sauce

SEASONINGS

Chili Powder
Cinnamon
Cumin
Curry Powder
Italian seasoning
Oregano

Recipe Key

There are graphic icons on recipes pages. Use this key to understand what each graphic means:

 Recipe Preparation Time

 Vegetarian Recipe

 Kid's Favorite

 All nutritional information for this recipe does NOT include the Pita Pocket since the quantity consumed varies by recipe and meal plan. A standard one-half 6" pita pocket has approximately 80-90 calories each. Please refer to the food label on the pita packaging to get an accurate count. If you follow the Pocket Diet Meal Plan, you do not have to keep track of your calories as long as you stay within the plan's recommendations

Recipe Index

	Prep Time	Kids	Vegetarian	Page
CHICKEN STRIP POCKETS				
Chicken Strip Pita	5			102
Chicken Ranch Pita	5	X		102
Chicken Club Pita	5	X		103
Chicken Parmegiana Pita	5			103
Honey Mustard Chicken Strip	5	X		104
BBQ Chicken Strip Pita	5	X		104
CHINESE POCKETS				
Moo Shoo Chicken Pockets	15			106
Chinese Chicken Salad	5			106
Pita Stickers	15			107
Peking Pockets	10			108
Egg Foo Yung Pockets	15			108
Teriyaki Beef	10			109
DELI FAVORITES				
BLT	5			112
Philly Cheese Steak Pocket	15			112
Croque Monsieur	10			113
Rueben	5			113
Pastrami & Pickles	5			114
Tuna Melt	10			114
Not So Sloppy Joe Pockets	5	X		115
Veggie Pita	5		X	115
DESSERT OMELETS				
Creamy Blueberry Omelet	10			118
Peach Ricotta Omelet	10			118
Blackberry Bramble Omelet	10			119
Strawberry Surprise Omelet	10			119
Cheesecake Omelet	10			120

	Prep Time	Kids	Vegetarian	Page
KABOBS				
Souvlaki w/ Tzatziki	15			182
Tzatziki	5			182
Raita	5			183
Beef Kabobs w/Tomato Salad	40			183
Tomato Salad	5			184
Asian Kabobs w/ Cucumber Salad	40			184
Cucumber Salad	5			185
Ham Kabobs	10			185
Garden Kabobs	10			186
Tikka w Cucumber Raita	40			186
Shrimp Kabobs	15			187
MEXICAN POCKETS				
Mexican Empanada	20			190
Sopapillas	10			190
Nachos	10			191
Tostadas	10			191
Chicken Fajita	30			192
Beef Fajita	30			193
PEANUT BUTTER PITAS				
PBJ	5	X	X	196
Grilled PBJ	5	X	X	196
PB & Bacon	5	X		197
Grilled Cheese & PB	5	X		197
PB & Applesause	5	X	X	198
PB & Apple	5	X	X	198
FlufferNutter	5	X	X	199
PB & Nutella	5	X	X	199
Peanut Butter & Banana	5	X	X	200

	Prep Time	Kids	Vegetarian	Page
QUESADILLA POCKETS				
Steak Quesadilla	10			220
BBQ Chicken Quesadilla	10			220
Krab Quesadilla	10			221
SHRIMP				
Shrimp Scampi	10			224
Southern Shrimp	10			224
Shrimp Po' Boy	15			225
Dill Shrimp	15			225
Shrimp & Avocado	15			226
Spicy Shrimp Salad	5			226
TAKE OUT INSPIRED				
Egg McPita	5			230
Fish Stick Pita	5			230
Club House Pita	5			231
TUNA POCKETS				
Traditional Tuna Salad	5			234
Twisted Tuna Salad	5			234
Tuna Salad Supreme	5			235
Tuna Tarragon Salad	5			235
Fancy Pants Tuna Salad	5			236
Crunchy Tuna Salad	5			236
Tangy Tuna Salad	5			237
Orange Tuna Salad	5			237
Herb Tuna Salad	5			238
Mexican Tuna Salad	5			238
Cheesy Tuna Salad	5			239
Apple Walnut Tuna	5			239
Tuna & Cannelloni Salad	5			240

burgers

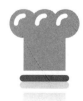

Pocket Chef Jenna Says...

Did you know that at restaurants men order burgers more than any other item? They work perfectly into the Pocket Diet plan. If you have a George Foreman grill, putting together a pita burger takes less time than it does to find your keys, let alone make it through the drive-thru!

Basic Burger Pocket

Time: 5 minutes
Servings: 1

Ingredients
  2 pita halves
  1 hamburger patty, cooked & halved
  2 lettuce leaves
  2 tomato slices
  2 onion slices
  2 pickle slices
  2 T ketchup
  2 t mustard

Spread the inside of pita halves with ketchup and mustard. Layer in lettuce, tomato, onion & pickle. Place burger half into pita & serve.

Nutritional Information (per serving)
Calories: 470, Total Fat: 17g, Saturated Fat: 5g, Cholesterol: 60mg, Sodium: 1200mg, Carbohydrates: 50g, Fiber: 12g, Sugar: 9g, Protein: 29g

Basic Veggie Burger Pocket

Time: 5 minutes
Servings: 1

Ingredients
  2 pita halves
  1 veggie burger patty, cooked & halved (Gardenburger)
  2 lettuce leaves
  2 tomato slices
  2 onion slices
  2 pickle slices
  2 T ketchup
  2 t mustard

Spread the inside of pita halves with ketchup and mustard. Layer in lettuce, tomato, onion & pickle. Place burger half into pita & serve.

Nutritional Information (per serving)
CALORIES: 380, TOTAL FAT: 5G, SATURATED FAT: 1G, CHOLESTEROL: 10MG, SODIUM: 1090MG, CARBOHYDRATES: 67G, FIBER: 16G, SUGAR: 10G, PROTEIN: 17G

Cheeseburger Pita

Time: 5 minutes
Servings 1

Ingredients
    2 pita halves
    1 hamburger patty, cooked & halved
    2 slices reduced fat cheddar cheese
    2 lettuce leaves
    2 tomato slices
    2 onion slices
    2 pickle slices
    2 T ketchup
    2 t mustard

Spread the inside of pita halves with ketchup and mustard. Layer in lettuce, tomato, onion & pickle. Place burger half & cheese into pita & serve.

Nutritional Information (per serving)
CALORIES: 560, TOTAL FAT: 20G, SATURATED FAT: 8G, CHOLESTEROL: 70MG, SODIUM: 1600MG, CARBOHYDRATES: 51G, FIBER: 11G, SUGAR: 11G, PROTEIN: 41G

BBQ Bacon Burger

Time: 5 minutes
Servings 1

Ingredients
    2 pita halves
    1 hamburger patty, cooked & halved
    2 slices reduced fat cheddar cheese
    2 lettuce leaves
    2 slices bacon, halved
    2 onion rings
    2 T BBQ sauce

Spread the inside of pita halves with BBQ sauce. Layer in lettuce, bacon & onion rings. Place burger half & cheese into pita & serve.

Nutritional Information (per serving)
CALORIES: 670, TOTAL FAT: 28G, SATURATED FAT: 11G, CHOLESTEROL: 80MG SODIUM: 1790MG, CARBOHYDRATES: 55G, FIBER: 9G, SUGAR: 14G, PROTEIN: 45G

Mushroom Swiss Burger Pocket

Time: 10 minutes
Servings: 1

Ingredients

2 pita halves
4 mushrooms, sliced
2 t balsamic vinegar
2 T light mayonnaise
1 burger patty, grilled and halved
1 slice Swiss cheese
2 lettuce leaves
4 tomato slices

Spritz a small non-stick skillet with cooking spray and heat to medium-high. Add mushrooms and sauté until soft, about 2 minutes. In a small bowl combine mayonnaise and balsamic vinegar. Spread mayonnaise mixture inside pita halves. Arrange remaining ingredients inside & serve.

Nutritional Information (per serving)

CALORIES: 350, TOTAL FAT: 23G, SATURATED FAT: 9G, CHOLESTEROL: 75MG, SODIUM: 810MG, CARBOHYDRATES: 9G, FIBER: 2G, SUGAR: 5G, PROTEIN: 26G

caesar salad
pockets

Pocket Chef Jenna Says...

In the refrigerated section of your produce department you'll find a number of bagged Caesar Salad kits. Most contain lettuce, dressing, cheese and croutons, and will fill 6-8 pitas. Look for the light versions, which have lower fat dressings and omit the cheese and/or croutons.

Caesar Salad Pockets

Time: 5 minutes
Servings: 6

Ingredients
1 Caesar Salad kit
6 pita halves

Prepare kit according to package directions. Fill pitas & serve.

Nutritional Information (per serving)
CALORIES: 170, TOTAL FAT: 7G, SATURATED FAT: 1.5G, CHOLESTEROL: 5MG, SODIUM: 360MG, CARBOHYDRATES: 20G, FIBER: 5G, SUGAR: 2G, PROTEIN: 5G

Grilled Chicken Caesar Pockets

Time: 5 minutes
Servings: 6

Ingredients
1 Caesar Salad kit
1 (6 oz) prepared chicken strips or one grilled chicken breast, sliced
6 pita halves

Prepare kit according to package directions. Mix in chicken strips. Fill pitas & serve.

Nutritional Information (per serving)
CALORIES: 210, TOTAL FAT: 8G, SATURATED FAT: 2G, CHOLESTEROL: 30MG, SODIUM: 380MG, CARBOHYDRATES: 20G, FIBER: 5G, SUGAR: 2G, PROTEIN: 13G

Shrimp Caesar Salad Pockets

Time: 5 minutes
Servings: 6

Ingredients
1 Caesar Salad kit
1 cup cooked cocktail shrimp
6 pita halves

Prepare kit according to package directions. Mix in shrimp. Fill pitas & serve.

Nutritional Information (per serving)
CALORIES: 200, TOTAL FAT: 7G, SATURATED FAT: 1.5G, CHOLESTEROL: 35MG, SODIUM: 530MG, CARBOHYDRATES: 23G, FIBER: 5G, SUGAR: 4G, PROTEIN: 9G

Mexican Caesar Salad Pockets

Time: 10 minutes
Servings: 6

Ingredients
1 Caesar Salad kit
1 T lime juice
¼ t chili powder
1 avocado, cubed
1 tomato, seeded and iced
¼ cup frozen corn, thawed
6 pita halves

In a large bowl mix Caesar dressing with lime and chili powder. Toss with remaining **ingredients**. Fill pitas & serve.

Nutritional Information (per serving)
CALORIES: 230, TOTAL FAT: 12G, SATURATED FAT: 2.5G, CHOLESTEROL: 5MG, SODIUM: 370MG, CARBOHYDRATES: 25G, FIBER: 7G, SUGAR: 3G, PROTEIN: 6G

calzone
pockets

Pocket Chef Jenna Says...

Pitas are remarkably like the bread that holds calzone filling, without the all-day prep. Heat up the filling in the microwave, stuff into warm pita pockets, top with a spoonful or two of prepared marinara, and voila – you are a gourmet Italian chef. Amazing really, why did no one think of this before the Pocket Diet?

Broccoli Pockets

Time: 10 minutes
Servings: 4

Ingredients

4 pita pockets (1/2 each)
1 package frozen broccoli, thawed, drained, & chopped
1 t bottled minced garlic
1 cup reduced fat mozzarella shredded
¼ cup parmesan
¼ cup bottled roasted red peppers, chopped
1 t oregano

Combine all ingredients in a microwave safe bowl. Heat for one minute, stir, heat for another minute. Fill pitas. Place stuffed pitas on a plate and microwave for one minute more.

Nutritional Information (per serving)

CALORIES: 210, TOTAL FAT: 7G, SATURATED FAT: 4.5G, CHOLESTEROL: 20MG, SODIUM: 420MG, CARBOHYDRATES: 22G, FIBER: 6G, SUGAR: 3G, PROTEIN: 16G

Spinach Artichoke Calzone

Time: 10 minutes
Servings: 6

Ingredients

6 pita pockets (1/2 each)
1 package frozen spinach, thawed, drained, & chopped
1 can artichokes, drained and chopped
1 T bottled minced garlic
1 cup fat free mozzarella
1 cup fat free ricotta
¼ cup parmesan
Pinch nutmeg

Combine all ingredients in a microwave safe bowl. Heat for one minute, stir, heat for another minute. Fill pitas. Place stuffed pitas on a plate and microwave for one minute more. Serve with prepared marinara for dipping.

Nutritional Information (per serving)

CALORIES: 220, TOTAL FAT: 5G, SATURATED FAT: 3G, CHOLESTEROL: 20MG, SODIUM: 510MG, CARBOHYDRATES: 26G, FIBER: 8G, SUGAR: 2G, PROTEIN: 18G

Sausage Calzone

Time: 10 minutes
Servings: 6

Ingredients

    6 pita pockets (1/2 each)
    ¼ cup Pita-za sauce or pizza sauce
    8 oz veggie sausage patties, cooked and chopped (Morningstar Farms)
    ¼ cup bottled roasted red pepper, chopped
    1 small can sliced mushrooms, drained
    1 T bottled minced garlic
    1 cups fat free ricotta
    ¼ cup parmesan
    1 T parsley, chopped
    Pinch nutmeg

Combine all ingredients in a microwave safe bowl. Heat for one minute, stir, heat for another minute. Spread pita's with 1 T Pita-za sauce. Spoon filling into Pitas. Place stuffed pitas on a plate and microwave for one minute more. Serve with prepared marinara for dipping.

Nutritional Information (per serving)
CALORIES: 260, TOTAL FAT: 12G, SATURATED FAT: 6G, CHOLESTEROL: 20MG, SODIUM: 740MG, CARBOHYDRATES: 23G, FIBER: 5G, SUGAR: 2G, PROTEIN: 15G

Turkey Tomato Calzone

Time: 10 minutes
Servings: 6

Ingredients

    6 pita pockets (1/2 each)
    ½ pound cooked turkey breast, chopped
    3 sundried tomatoes, drained and chopped
    1 T bottled minced garlic
    1 cup fat free mozzarella
    1 cup fat free ricotta
    ¼ cup parmesan
    Pinch nutmeg

Combine all ingredients in a microwave safe bowl. Heat for one minute, stir, heat for another minute. Fill pitas. Place stuffed pitas on a plate and microwave for one minute more. Serve with prepared marinara for dipping.

Nutritional Information (per serving)
CALORIES: 250, TOTAL FAT: 8G, SATURATED FAT: 5G, CHOLESTEROL: 40MG, SODIUM: 900MG, CARBOHYDRATES: 23G, FIBER: 5G, SUGAR: 3G, PROTEIN: 22G

Seafood Calzone

10

Time: 10 minutes
Servings: 6

Ingredients
6 pita pockets (1/2 each)
¼ cup cooked shrimp, chopped
¼ cup crab, or krab
1 T bottled minced garlic
2 green onions, chopped
1 cups fat free mozzarella
1 cups fat free ricotta
¼ cup parmesan
1 T oregano, chopped
Pinch nutmeg

Combine all ingredients in a microwave safe bowl. Heat for one minute, stir, heat for another minute. Fill pitas. Place stuffed pitas on a plate and microwave for one minute more. Serve with prepared marinara for dipping.

Nutritional Information (per serving)
CALORIES: 260, TOTAL FAT: 8G, SATURATED FAT: 5G, CHOLESTEROL: 70MG, SODIUM: 570MG, CARBOHYDRATES: 23G, FIBER: 4G, SUGAR: 2G, PROTEIN: 22G

Ham and Spinach Calzone

Time: 10 minutes
Servings: 6

Ingredients
6 pita pockets (1/2 each)
4 oz turkey ham lunchmeat, chopped
1 package frozen spinach, thawed, drained, & chopped
¼ cup bottled roasted red peppers, chopped
1 T bottled minced garlic
1 cups fat free mozzarella
1 cups fat free ricotta
¼ cup parmesan
Pinch nutmeg

Combine all ingredients in a microwave safe bowl. Heat for one minute, stir, heat for another minute. Fill pitas. Place stuffed pitas on a plate and microwave for one minute more.

Nutritional Information (per serving)
CALORIES: 250, TOTAL FAT: 9G, SATURATED FAT: 5G, CHOLESTEROL: 35MG, SODIUM: 660MG, CARBOHYDRATES: 23G, FIBER: 6G, SUGAR: 2G, PROTEIN: 20G

cheese
pocket fillings

Pocket Chef Jenna Says...

Cheese sandwiches are a Southern thing. Kind of like a guilty pleasure...They work well in pitas, especially for picnics. For the kiddos, a hint would be to wrap the pitas in paper towels (they don't fit in sandwich bags). If the filling might run out Use a lettuce leaf and tuck it around the filling.

Cheesy Salad Pocket

Time: 15 minutes
Servings: 6

Ingredients

2 small cucumbers; peeled & diced
2 small tomato; diced
1 small red onion; diced
1/2 red bell pepper; diced
1/2 green bell pepper; diced
4 T salad dressing (your choice); low fat
3 T cheddar cheese; shredded & low fat
1/4 cup alfalfa sprouts (optional)

Combine all ingredients into a bowl. Salt & pepper to taste. Fill pocket & serve.

Nutritional Information (per serving)

CALORIES: 56, TOTAL FAT: 1G, SATURATED FAT: 0G, CHOLESTEROL 0MG, SODIUM: 117MG, CARBOHYDRATES: 10G, FIBER: 2G, SUGAR: 5G, PROTEIN: 2G

 This recipe does not include nutritional information for the pita pocket bread. For this nutritional information, go to page 71.

Pimento Cheddar Pockets

Time: 5 minutes
Servings: 4

Ingredients

¼ cup jarred pimentos, drained and chopped
1 cup reduced fat cheddar, shredded
¼ cup light mayonnaise
¼ cup fat free cream cheese
1 T parsley, chopped
salt & pepper

In a small bowl combine mayonnaise and cream cheese. Stir in remaining ingredients. Fill pitas & serve.

Nutritional Information (per serving)

CALORIES: 170, TOTAL FAT: 14G, SATURATED FAT: 6G, CHOLESTEROL: 30MG, SODIUM: 370MG, CARBOHYDRATES: 2G, FIBER: 0G, SUGAR: 0G, PROTEIN: 9G

 This recipe does not include nutritional information for the pita pocket bread. For this nutritional information, go to page 71.

Monterey Jack and Jalapeno

Time: 5 minutes
Servings: 4

Ingredients
4 pita halves
1 cup Monterey jack cheese, shredded
1 T pickled jalapeno peppers, chopped
¼ cup light mayonnaise
¼ cup fat free cream cheese
1 T green onions, chopped
salt & pepper

In a small bowl combine mayonnaise and cream cheese. Stir in remaining ingredients. Fill pitas & serve.

Nutritional Information (per serving)

CALORIES: 330, TOTAL FAT: 17G, SATURATED FAT: 4G, CHOLESTEROL: 10MG, SODIUM: 880MG, CARBOHYDRATES: 18G, FIBER: 7G, SUGAR: 5G, PROTEIN: 26G

 This recipe does not include nutritional information for the pita pocket bread. For this nutritional information, go to page 71.

Feta Tomato Pockets

Time: 5 minutes
Servings: 4

Ingredients

1 cup crumbled feta
1 tomato, seeded & chopped
¼ cup basil, chopped
¼ cup light mayonnaise
¼ cup fat free cream cheese
salt & pepper

In a small bowl combine mayonnaise and cream cheese. Stir in remaining ingredients. Fill pitas & serve.

Nutritional Information (per serving)

CALORIES: 170, TOTAL FAT: 13G, SATURATED FAT: 6G, CHOLESTEROL: 40MG, SODIUM: 610MG, CARBOHYDRATES: 5G, FIBER: 0G, SUGAR: 2G, PROTEIN: 8G

 This recipe does not include nutritional information for the pita pocket bread. For this nutritional information, go to page 71.

Italian Cheese & Sundried Tomatoes Pockets

Time: 5 minutes
Servings: 4

Ingredients

1 cup reduced fat mozzarella, shredded
1 T Parmesan
1 T sundried tomatoes, chopped
¼ cup basil, chopped
¼ cup light mayonnaise
¼ cup fat free cream cheese
salt & pepper

In a small bowl combine mayonnaise and cream cheese. Stir in remaining ingredients. Fill pitas & serve.

Nutritional Information (per serving)

CALORIES: 150, TOTAL FAT: 11G, SATURATED FAT: 4G, CHOLESTEROL: 25MG, SODIUM: 380MG, CARBOHYDRATES: 3G, FIBER: 0G, SUGAR: 0G, PROTEIN: 11G

 This recipe does not include nutritional information for the pita pocket bread. For this nutritional information, go to page 71.

Creamy Cheese & Vegetable Pockets

Time: 5 minutes
Servings: 2

Ingredients

½ cup light Cream Cheese
¼ cup light Sour cream
1 Celery, minced
1 Carrot, grated
1 Radish, minced
1 Green onion, chopped
Dash of Worcestershire sauce

In a small bowl combine cream cheese and sour cream. Stir in remaining ingredients. Fill pitas & serve.

Nutritional Information (per serving)

CALORIES: 140, TOTAL FAT: 8G, SATURATED FAT: 5G, CHOLESTEROL: 30MG, SODIUM: 260MG, CARBOHYDRATES: 9G, FIBER: 2G, SUGAR: 7G, PROTEIN: 9G

 This recipe does not include nutritional information for the pita pocket bread. For this nutritional information, go to page 71.

chicken strip
pockets

Pocket Chef Jenna Says...

There are few foods kids love more than chicken strips. Fast and easy, they are a parents friend too. (Use strips or nuggets for these pitas, whatever you have on hand. Vegetarian "chicken" nuggets work too)

Chicken Strip Pita

Time: 5 minutes
Servings: 1

Ingredients
1 pita half
2 chicken strips or 3 nuggets, cooked
1 T light mayonnaise
2 tomato slices
2 dill pickle slices
¼ cup shredded lettuce

Spread inside of pita with mayonnaise. Fill with remaining ingredients & serve.

Nutritional Information (per serving)
CALORIES: 280, TOTAL FAT: 15G, SATURATED FAT: 3G, CHOLESTEROL: 15MG, SODIUM: 710MG, CARBOHYDRATES: 26G, FIBER: 5G, SUGAR: 3G, PROTEIN: 11G

Chicken Ranch Pita

Time: 5 minutes
Servings: 1

Ingredients
1 pita half
2 chicken strips or 3 nuggets, cooked
1 T light ranch
2 tomato slices
¼ cup shredded lettuce

Spread inside of pita with ranch. Fill with remaining ingredients & serve.

Nutritional Information (per serving)
CALORIES: 320, TOTAL FAT: 19G, SATURATED FAT: 3.5G, CHOLESTEROL: 20MG, SODIUM: 580MG, CARBOHYDRATES: 25G, FIBER: 5G, SUGAR: 3G, PROTEIN: 11G

Chicken Club Pita

Time: 5 minutes
Servings: 1

Ingredients
1 pita half
2 chicken strips or 3 nuggets, cooked
1 T light mayonnaise
1 slice reduced fat Swiss cheese
1 slice turkey ham lunchmeat
2 tomato slices
¼ cup shredded lettuce

Spread inside of pita with mayonnaise. Fill with remaining ingredients & serve.

Nutritional Information (per serving)
CALORIES: 420, TOTAL FAT: 21G, SATURATED FAT: 7G, CHOLESTEROL: 65MG, SODIUM: 850MG, CARBOHYDRATES: 27G, FIBER: 6G, SUGAR: 3G, PROTEIN: 28G

Chicken Parmegiana Pita

Time: 5 minutes
Servings: 1

Ingredients
1 pita half
2 chicken strips or 3 nuggets, cooked
1 T Pita-za sauce, or 1 T prepared marinara sauce
½ slice Provolone cheese

Spread inside of pita with sauce. Arrange cheese and strips inside. Microwave 30 seconds, or until cheese melts & serve.

Nutritional Information (per serving)
CALORIES: 310, TOTAL FAT: 17G, SATURATED FAT: 6G, CHOLESTEROL: 40MG, SODIUM: 760MG, CARBOHYDRATES: 24G, FIBER: 5G, SUGAR: 2G, PROTEIN: 16G

Honey Mustard Chicken Strip

Time: 5 minutes
Serves 1

Ingredients
1 pita half
2 chicken strips or 3 nuggets, cooked
1 T honey mustard dressing
2 tomato slices
¼ cup shredded lettuce

Spread inside of pita with dressing. Fill with remaining ingredients & serve.

Nutritional Information (per serving)
CALORIES: 250, TOTAL FAT: 9G, SATURATED FAT: 2.5G, CHOLESTEROL: 20MG, SODIUM: 430MG, CARBOHYDRATES: 31G, FIBER: 5G, SUGAR: 9G, PROTEIN: 10G

BBQ Chicken Strip Pita

Time: 5 minutes
Serves 1

Ingredients
1 pita half
2 chicken strips or 3 nuggets, cooked
1 T BBQ sauce
2 tomato slices
¼ cup shredded lettuce

Spread inside of pita with BBQ sauce. Fill with remaining ingredients & serve.

Nutritional Information (per serving)
CALORIES: 220, TOTAL FAT: 6G, SATURATED FAT: 2G, CHOLESTEROL: 20MG, SODIUM: 560MG, CARBOHYDRATES: 29G, FIBER: 5G, SUGAR: 7G, PROTEIN: 10G

chinese
pockets

Pocket Chef Jenna Says...

Asian foods are generally very healthy, it's the Americanized versions that get us into trouble. These healthy options should curb your yearning to order in, and help whittle your waistline.

Moo Shoo Chicken Pockets

Time: 15 minutes
Servings 4-6

Ingredients
2 egg whites
½ pound ground chicken
2 t vegetable oil
1 garlic clove, minced
½ t ground ginger
2 cups shredded cabbage (coleslaw mix)
½ cup chopped zucchini
2 green onions, sliced
¼ cup Hoisin sauce

Heat a nonstick skillet over medium high heat. Spray with cooking spray and add egg whites. Cook until done. Remove and cut into strips. Add oil to pan. Cook chicken garlic and ginger until crumbly. Add vegetables. Cook 3 minutes, or until tender. Stir in hoisin & egg strips. Fill pitas & serve

Nutritional Information (per serving)
CALORIES: 150, TOTAL FAT: 0G, SATURATED FAT: 0G, CHOLESTEROL: 0MG, SODIUM: 340MG, CARBOHYDRATES: 12G, FIBER: 2G, SUGAR: 1G, PROTEIN: 14G

 This recipe does not include nutritional information for the pita pocket bread. For this nutritional information, go to page 71.

Chinese Chicken Salad

Time: 5 minutes
Servings 2

Ingredients
1 T oil
2 t cider vinegar
1 t sesame oil
1 T honey
pinch ginger
pinch sesame seeds
1T peanut butter
4 oz chicken breast, cooked and sliced
¼ cup red pepper strips
2 green onions, chopped

In a small bowl combine dressing ingredients (oil through peanut butter). Toss with chicken and vegetables. Fill pitas & serve.

Nutritional Information (per serving)
CALORIES: 310, TOTAL FAT: 18G, SATURATED FAT: 3G, CHOLESTEROL: 50MG, SODIUM: 60MG, CARBOHYDRATES: 20G, FIBER: 4G, SUGAR: 13G, PROTEIN: 21G

Pita Stickers

Time: 15 minutes
Servings 4

Ingredients
½ pound ground turkey
2 T water chestnuts, chopped
1 green onion, chopped
2 t soy sauce
pinch ground ginger
pinch red pepper flake
1 t honey
2 T rice vinegar
1 cucumber, peeled, seeded, sliced
1 carrot, grated
4 T Hoisin sauce

In a small bowl combine turkey, water chestnuts, green onion, soy, ginger & pepper flake. Form into 4 patties. Heat a non-stick pan over medium-high heat. Coat with cooking spray and add patties. Cook 3 minutes on each side, or until cooked through. While cooking, combine honey, rice vinegar, cucumber and carrot. Spread inside of pita with 1 T Hoisin. Add cooked patty & fill with cucumber salad & serve.

Nutritional Information (per serving)
CALORIES: 200, TOTAL FAT: 8G, SATURATED FAT: 2G, CHOLESTEROL: 60MG, SODIUM: 550MG, CARBOHYDRATES: 15G, FIBER: 2G, SUGAR: 5G, PROTEIN: 18G

 This recipe does not include nutritional information for the pita pocket bread. For this nutritional information, go to page 71.

Peking Pockets

Time: 10 minutes
Servings 4

Ingredients
½ cup Hoisin sauce
1 T soy
1 T honey
1 T rice vinegar
pinch ginger
1 t minced garlic, bottled
½ pound boneless, skinless chicken breast
4 green onions, chopped

In a small bowl combine sauce (Hoisin through garlic). Remove two tablespoons and reserve the rest. Marinade chicken in 2 T sauce. Heat a non-stick pan over medium-high heat. Coat with cooking spray and add chicken. Cook 3 minutes each side, or until cooked through. Shred with a fork and add to reserved sauce. Fill pitas & top with green onions & serve.

Nutritional Information (per serving)
CALORIES: 260, TOTAL FAT: 6G, SATURATED FAT: 1.5G, CHOLESTEROL: 50MG, SODIUM: 910MG, CARBOHYDRATES: 32G, FIBER: 5G, SUGAR: 10G, PROTEIN: 22G

 This recipe does not include nutritional information for the pita pocket bread. For this nutritional information, go to page 71.

Egg Foo Yung Pockets

Time: 15 minutes
Servings 8

Ingredients
3/4 cup egg substitute – or 1 egg, 4 egg whites
1 cup cooked salad shrimp
½ cup water chestnuts, chopped
½ cup bean sprouts, chopped
¼ cup green onions, chopped
pinch of ginger
¼ cup prepared Chinese mustard or Plum Sauce

In a small bowl combine egg substitute, shrimp, vegetables and ginger. Heat a non-stick pan over medium-high heat. Coat with cooking spray. Cook 2-4 at a time, depending on the size of your pan. Spread inside of pita with mustard or Plum sauce. Slide in an egg foo yung & serve.

Nutritional Information (per serving)
CALORIES: 60, TOTAL FAT: .5G, SATURATED FAT: 12G, CHOLESTEROL: 50MG, SODIUM: 90MG, CARBOHYDRATES: 5G, FIBER: 0G, SUGAR: 1G, PROTEIN: 4G

Teriyaki Beef

Time: 10 minutes
Servings 2

Ingredients
2 pita halves
¼ pound round steak, sliced thin
¼ cup sliced mushrooms
¼ cup red pepper strips
¼ cup onion, sliced
3 T prepared teriyaki sauce

Heat a non-stick pan over medium-high heat and coat with cooking spray and steak. When no longer pink add vegetables and cook one minute. Add Teriyaki sauce and cook 1 minute more. Fill pitas & serve.

Nutritional Information (per serving)
CALORIES: 140, TOTAL FAT: 3G, SATURATED FAT: 1G, CHOLESTEROL: 50MG, SODIUM: 1070MG, CARBOHYDRATES: 8G, FIBER: 0G, SUGAR: 4G, PROTEIN: 20G

deli
favorites

Pocket Chef Jenna Says...

Nothing is off limits, you only have to learn to control the portions of it. Craving the salty-sweet combo of a Croque Monsieur or the comfort of a Tuna Melt? Here's how to do it, without straying from your eating plan.

BLT

Time: 5 minutes
Servings 1

Ingredients
    1 pita half
    1 T light mayonnaise
    1 slice bacon, crumbled
    2 tomato slices
    1 lettuce leaf

Spread mayonnaise inside pita. Sprinkle bacon into pita. Place lettuce and tomato inside & serve.

Nutritional Information (per serving)
CALORIES: 260, TOTAL FAT: 18G, SATURATED FAT: 5MG, CHOLESTEROL: 20MG, SODIUM: 410MG, CARBOHYDRATES: 19G, FIBER: 5, SUGAR: 2G, PROTEIN: 5G

Philly Cheese Steak Pocket

Time: 15 minutes
Servings: 1

Ingredients
    1 pita half
    2 oz. beef tenderloin; 2 pieces sliced 1/2" thin
    1/2 green bell pepper; sliced into long strips
    1/2 small onion; sliced
    1 oz. provolone cheese; low fat
    1 T olive oil

Heat oil in skillet on med-high heat for 1 minute. Add meat; cook each side for 1 minute. Remove meat from pan on to a plate; top with cheese. Cover plate with lid of pan or another plate to keep meat warm. Add veggies to same pan; stir until tender. Salt & pepper to taste. Fill pocket & serve.

Nutritional Information (per serving)
CALORIES: 313, TOTAL FAT: 22G, SATURATED FAT: 9G, CHOLESTEROL: 56MG, SODIUM: 151MG, CARBOHYDRATES: 12G, FIBER: 3G, SUGAR: 4G, PROTEIN: 21G

Croque Monsieur

Time: 10 minutes
Servings 1

Ingredients
1 pita half
1 t Dijon mustard
1 t raspberry preserves
1 slice reduced fat Swiss cheese
1 slice turkey ham lunchmeat

Spread one side of pocket with mustard, the other side with preserves. Arrange the ham and cheese inside the pita Grill in a pan coated with cooking spray until cheese melts. (microwave if you're at work) & serve.

Nutritional Information (per serving)
CALORIES: 180, TOTAL FAT: 4G, SATURATED FAT: 1.5G, CHOLESTEROL: 35MG, SODIUM: 658MG, CARBOHYDRATES: 21G, FIBER: 4G, SUGAR: 3G, PROTEIN: 9G

Rueben

Time: 5 minutes
Serves 1

Ingredients
1 pita half
1 T reduced fat mayonnaise
2 slices corned beef lunchmeat
1 slice reduced fat Swiss cheese
2 T sauerkraut

Spread mayonnaise inside pocket. Arrange corned beef, cheese, and sauerkraut. Grill in a pan coated with cooking spray until cheese melts. (microwave if you're at work) & serve.

Nutritional Information (per serving)
CALORIES: 330, TOTAL FAT: 16G, SATURATED FAT: 5G, CHOLESTEROL: 80MG, SODIUM: 1550MG, CARBOHYDRATES: 22G, FIBER: 5G, SUGAR: 4G, PROTEIN: 21G

Pastrami & Pickles

Time: 5 minutes
Servings 1

Ingredients
    1 pita half
    1 t butter, softened
    1 t grain mustard
    2 slices pastrami lunchmeat
    1 dill pickle, sliced lengthwise

Spread one side of pocket with mustard, the other with butter. Arrange pastrami and pickles inside pita. Grill in a pan coated with cooking spray until cheese melts. (microwave if you're at work) & serve.

Nutritional Information (per serving)
CALORIES: 210, TOTAL FAT: 7G, SATURATED FAT: 3.5MG, CHOLESTEROL: 40MG, SODIUM: 1680MG, CARBOHYDRATES: 21G, FIBER: 5G, SUGAR: 3G, PROTEIN: 14G

Tuna Melt

Time: 10 minutes
Servings 1

Ingredients
    1 pita half
    1 slice reduced fat cheddar
    3 T tuna salad

Stuff pocket with tuna salad and cheese. Grill in a pan coated with cooking spray until cheese melts. (microwave if you're at work) & serve.

Nutritional Information (per serving)
CALORIES: 200, TOTAL FAT: 6G, SATURATED FAT: 2MG, CHOLESTEROL: 10MG, SODIUM: 470MG, CARBOHYDRATES: 20G, FIBER: 4G, SUGAR: 3G, PROTEIN: 16G

Not So Sloppy Joe Pockets

Time: 5 minutes
Servings: 4

Ingredients

4 pita halves
12 oz. ground sirloin (90% lean)
1/2 cup green pepper; diced
1/2 cup onion; diced
1/2 cup celery; diced
1 Tbsp. canola oil
1 cup of sloppy joe sauce (your choice)

Heat oil in large skillet on medium heat. Add veggies and sauté for 2 minutes. Add meat and brown meat for 5 minutes. Add sauce; turn heat to low and simmer for 10 minutes. Fill pocket & serve.

Nutritional Information (per serving)

CALORIES: 199, TOTAL FAT: 11G, SATURATED FAT: 4G, CHOLESTEROL: 32MG, SODIUM: 500MG, CARBOHYDRATES: 13G, FIBER: 1G, SUGAR: 9G, PROTEIN: 12G

Veggie Pita

Time: 5 minutes
Serves 1

Ingredients

1 pita half
2 T light cream cheese
1 lettuce leaf
2 cucumber slices
2 tomato slices
2 green pepper strips
1 onion slice

Spread cream cheese inside pita. Fill with vegetables & serve.

Nutritional Information (per serving)

CALORIES: 170, TOTAL FAT: 5G, SATURATED FAT: 3.5G, CHOLESTEROL: 15MG, SODIUM: 300MG, CARBOHYDRATES: 23G, FIBER: 5G, SUGAR: 6G, PROTEIN: 7G

dessert
omelets

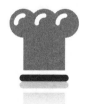

Pocket Chef Jenna Says...

Sometimes you need something a little sweet, a little special to start the day off right. Try these tasty treats next time you feel like indulging...at breakfast! (frozen fruit is always available, use fresh when in season).

Creamy Blueberry Omelet

Time: 10 minutes
Servings: 1

Ingredients

  1 pita half
  1 egg
  1 egg white
  1 packet no-cal sweetener (Splenda)
  1 T light cream cheese
  1 t vanilla
  12 frozen blueberries

In a small bowl combine eggs, sweetener, cream cheese and vanilla. Coat a small non-stick pan with butter flavored cooking spray and place over medium heat. Add mixture to pan. When bottom sets, scatter berries over the top. When the sides are set, about two minutes, flip over for another minute. Fill pitas & serve.

Nutritional Information (per serving)

CALORIES: 175, TOTAL FAT: 5G, SATURATED FAT: 2G, CHOLESTEROL: 180MG, SODIUM: 160MG, CARBOHYDRATES: 19G, FIBER: 1G, SUGAR: 15G, PROTEIN: 10G

Peach Ricotta Omelet

Time: 10 minutes
Servings: 1

Ingredients

  1 pita half
  1 egg
  1 egg white
  1 packet no-cal sweetener (Splenda)
  1 T fat free ricotta cheese
  ½ t almond extract
  4 frozen peach slices

In a small bowl combine eggs, sweetener, ricotta cheese and almond extract. Coat a small non-stick pan with butter flavored cooking spray and place over medium heat. Arrange peach slices in pan, pour mixture over the top. When the sides are set, about two minutes, flip over for another minute. Fill pitas & serve.

CALORIES: 190, TOTAL FAT: 7G, SATURATED FAT: 3.5G, CHOLESTEROL: 220MG, SODIUM: 180MG, CARBOHYDRATES: 17G, FIBER: 1G, SUGAR: 15G, PROTEIN: 12G

Blackberry Bramble Omelet

Time: 10 minutes
Servings: 1

Ingredients
    1 pita half
    1 egg
    1 egg white
    1 packet no-cal sweetener (Splenda)
    1 T light cream cheese
    1 t vanilla
    1 pinch nutmeg
    12 frozen blackberries

In a small bowl combine eggs, sweetener, cream cheese, nutmeg, and vanilla. Coat a small non-stick pan with butter flavored cooking spray and place over medium heat. Add mixture to pan. When bottom sets, scatter berries over the top. When the sides are set, about two minutes, flip over for another minute. Fill pitas & serve.

Nutritional Information (per serving)
CALORIES: 210, TOTAL FAT: 7G, SATURATED FAT: 2.5G, CHOLESTEROL: 220MG, SODIUM: 170MG, CARBOHYDRATES: 21G, FIBER: 6G, SUGAR: 14G, PROTEIN: 13G

Strawberry Surprise Omelet

Time: 10 minutes
Servings: 1

Ingredients
    1 pita half
    1 egg
    1 egg white
    1 packet no-cal sweetener (Splenda)
    1 T light cream cheese
    1 t vanilla
    4 fresh strawberries, sliced
    1 T sugar free strawberry jam

In a small bowl combine eggs, sweetener, cream cheese and vanilla. Coat a small non-stick pan with butter flavored cooking spray and place over medium heat. Add mixture to pan. When the sides are set, about two minutes, flip over for another minute. Spread jam inside pitas. Arrange berries over jam. Add omelet & serve.

Nutritional Information (per serving)
CALORIES: 190, TOTAL FAT: 6G, SATURATED FAT: 2.5G, CHOLESTEROL: 220MG, SODIUM: 180MG, CARBOHYDRATES: 19G, FIBER: 1G, SUGAR: 12G, PROTEIN: 12G

Cheesecake Omelet

Time: 10 minutes
Servings: 1

Ingredients
1 pita half
1 egg
1 egg white
1 packet no-cal sweetener (Splenda)
1 T light cream cheese
1 T fat free ricotta cheese
1 t vanilla
1 T sugar free raspberry jam

In a small bowl combine eggs, sweetener, cheeses and vanilla. Coat a small non-stick pan with butter flavored cooking spray and place over medium heat. Add mixture to pan. When the sides are set, about two minutes, flip over for another minute. Spread jam inside pitas. Add omelet & serve.

Nutritional Information (per serving)
CALORIES: 210, TOTAL FAT: 8G, SATURATED FAT: 3.5G, CHOLESTEROL: 225MG, SODIUM: 230MG, CARBOHYDRATES: 17G, FIBER: 0G, SUGAR: 15G, PROTEIN: 13G

egg pockets

Pocket Chef Jenna Says...

Protein really helps curb the appetite, and egg whites are a great source. Besides, don't these recipes sound yummy?

Egg McPita

Time: 5 minutes
Servings: 1

Ingredients
  1 pita half
  1 egg
  1 slice reduced fat American cheese
  1 slice turkey ham lunchmeat

Heat a small non-stick pan over medium-high heat. Spray with cooking spray and crack egg into pan. Cook until bottom is set, about 1 minute, then flip and cook until desired doneness. Arrange in pita with ham & cheese.

Nutritional Information (per serving)
CALORIES: 280, TOTAL FAT: 13G, SATURATED FAT: 6G, CHOLESTEROL: 305MG
SODIUM: 750MG, CARBOHYDRATES: 18G, FIBER: 4G, SUGAR: 3G, PROTEIN: 21G

Ham, Egg & Cheese Pocket

Time: 5 minutes
Servings: 1

Ingredients
  1 pita half
  1/3 cup egg whites
  1/4 cup lean ham; diced
  2 T cheddar or Monterey Jack cheese; low fat & shredded

Coat skillet with nonstick cooking spray & place on medium heat. Warm ham for one minute. Add egg whites & cheese. Stir until firm. Salt & pepper to taste. Fill pocket & serve.

Nutritional Information (per serving)
CALORIES: 185, TOTAL FAT: 3G, SATURATED FAT: 1G, CHOLESTEROL: 20MG,
SODIUM: 892MG, CARBOHYDRATES: 19G, FIBER: 3G, SUGAR: 1, PROTEIN : 25G

Veggie Scramble Pocket

Time: 10 minutes
Servings: 1

Ingredients

- 1 pita half
- 1/3 cup egg whites
- 1/2 cup mixed bell peppers (red, green & yellow); diced
- 1/4 medium onion; diced
- 3 medium mushrooms; diced
- 2 T cheddar or Monterey Jack cheese; low fat & shredded

Coat skillet with nonstick cooking spray & place on medium heat. Sauté veggies for 3-4 minutes or until tender. Add eggs and cheese; stir until egg whites are firm. Salt & pepper to taste. Fill pocket & serve.

Nutritional Information (per serving)

CALORIES: 186, TOTAL FAT: 2G, SATURATED FAT: 1G, CHOLESTEROL: 3MG, SODIUM: 594MG, CARBOHYDRATES: 24G, FIBER: 3G, SUGAR: 5G, PROTEIN: 18G

Swiss Mushroom Egg Pocket

Time: 3 minutes
Servings: 1

Ingredients

- 1 pita half
- 1/3 cup egg whites
- 1/3 cup mushrooms, (your choice) chopped
- 2 T Swiss cheese; shredded & low fat
- 1 T parsley; chopped (optional)

Coat skillet with nonstick cooking spray; place on medium heat. Sauté mushrooms for 3-4 minutes or until tender. Add egg, cheese and parsley; stir until firm. Salt & pepper to taste. Fill pocket & serve.

Nutritional Information (per serving)

CALORIES: 154, TOTAL FAT: 1G, SATURATED FAT: TRACE, CHOLESTEROL: 5MG, SODIUM: 330MG, CARBOHYDRATES: 19G, FIBER: 2, SUGAR: 0G, PROTEIN: 16G

Broccoli Quiche Pocket

Time: 10 minutes
Servings: 1

Ingredients

- 1 pita half
- 1/3 cup egg whites
- 1/3 cup broccoli; chopped
- 2 Tbsp. cottage cheese; 1% fat
- 1 T onion; minced
- 1 T parmesan cheese; grated

Coat skillet with nonstick cooking spray & place on medium heat. Add onions & cook until soft. Mix egg & parmesan cheese in a bowl and cook for 1 minute. Then add broccoli & cottage cheese; stir lightly until eggs are firm. Salt & pepper to taste. Fill pocket & serve.

Nutritional Information (per serving)

CALORIES: 253, TOTAL FAT: 7G, SATURATED FAT: 1G, CHOLESTEROL: 60MG, SODIUM: 710MG, CARBOHYDRATES: 25G, FIBER: 3G, SUGAR: 3G, PROTEIN: 22G

Denver Scramble Pocket

Time: 5 minutes
Servings: 1

Ingredients

- 1 pita half
- 2 egg whites
- 1 slice turkey ham lunchmeat, chopped
- ¼ cup red pepper, chopped
- 2 T onion, chopped
- 2 T reduced fat cheddar cheese, shredded

Coat non-stick skillet with cooking spray and place over medium heat. Add all ingredients, stir until set, about 2 minutes. Fill pocket & serve.

Nutritional Information (per serving)

CALORIES: 110, TOTAL FAT: 2.5G, SATURATED FAT: 1G, CHOLESTEROL: 20MG, SODIUM: 400MG, CARBOHYDRATES: 5G, FIBER: 1G, SUGAR: 3G, PROTEIN: 16G

Herb Scramble Pocket

Time: 5 minutes
Servings: 1

Ingredients

1 pita half
3 egg whites
¼ cup fresh herbs, chopped (parsley, tarragon, chives, thyme)
2 T parmesan cheese, grated

Coat non-stick skillet with cooking spray and place over medium heat. Add all ingredients, stir until set, about 2 minutes. Fill pocket & serve.

Nutritional Information (per serving)

CALORIES: 120, TOTAL FAT: 4G, SATURATED FAT: 2.5G, CHOLESTEROL: 10MG, SODIUM: 400MG, CARBOHYDRATES: 3G, FIBER: 0G, SUGAR: 2G, PROTEIN: 16G

Huevos Rancheros Pockets

Time: 15 minutes
Servings: 4

Ingredients

4 pita halves
1 zucchini, chopped
1 red pepper, chopped
1 cup salsa
2 pitas, separated into four rounds
4 eggs
½ cup reduced fat cheddar cheese, shredded
2 t cilantro leaves

In a nonstick skillet coated with cooking spray sauté zucchini and pepper until they begin to brown. Add salsa and simmer 3 minutes. Break eggs into tomato mixture. Cover and cook 3 minutes, until eggs are done. Sprinkle with cheese. Spoon an egg and ¼ of tomato mixture onto each pita round. Sprinkle cilantro over, and serve.

Nutritional Information (per serving)

CALORIES: 130, TOTAL FAT: 6G, SATURATED FAT: 2G, CHOLESTEROL: 190MG, SODIUM: 590MG, CARBOHYDRATES: 11G, FIBER: 1G, SUGAR: 6G, PROTEIN: 10G

Mediterranean Egg Salad Pocket

Time: 5 minutes
Servings: 1

Ingredients

1 pita half
1 hard boiled egg; diced
2 T green bell pepper; diced
1 T olive oil
1 t onion; diced

Mix egg, veggies and oil in a small bowl. Salt & pepper to taste. Fill pocket & serve.

Nutritional Information (per serving)

CALORIES: 283, TOTAL FAT: 19G, SATURATED FAT: 3G, CHOLESTEROL: 212MG, SODIUM: 223MG, CARBOHYDRATES: 19G, FIBER: 1G, SUGAR: 1G, PROTEIN: 9G

Sausage Scramble Pocket

Time: 5 minutes
Servings: 1

Ingredients

1 pita half
2 egg whites
1 2 oz veggie sausage patty (Morning Star farms) thawed and chopped
1 t mustard
1 green onion chopped
2 T reduced fat cheddar cheese, shredded

Coat non-stick skillet with cooking spray and place over medium heat. Add all ingredients, stir until set, about 2 minutes. Fill pocket & serve.

Nutritional Information (per serving)

CALORIES: 330, TOTAL FAT: 17G, SATURATED FAT: 4G, CHOLESTEROL: 10MG, SODIUM: 880MG, CARBOHYDRATES: 18G, FIBER: 7G, SUGAR: 5G, PROTEIN: 26G

Sausage & Apple Scramble Pockets

Time: 5 minutes
Servings: 2

Ingredients
2 pita halves
2 egg whites
1 2 oz veggie sausage patty (Morning Star farms) thawed and chopped
¼ firm apple, chopped (Gala or Granny Smith)
1 pinch cinnamon
2 T reduced fat cheddar cheese, shredded

Coat non-stick skillet with cooking spray and place over medium heat. Add apple and sauté 2 minutes. Add remaining ingredients, stir until set, about 2 minutes. Fill pocket & serve.

Nutritional Information (per serving)
CALORIES: 140, TOTAL FAT: 4.5G, SATURATED FAT: .5G, CHOLESTEROL: 5MG, SODIUM: 450MG, CARBOHYDRATES: 8G, FIBER: 2G, SUGAR: 5G, PROTEIN: 16G

Spanish Scramble Pocket

Time: 5 minutes
Servings: 1

Ingredients
1 pita half
3 egg whites
¼ cup salsa
2 T reduced fat cheddar cheese, shredded

Coat non-stick skillet with cooking spray and place over medium heat. Add all ingredients, stir until set, about 2 minutes. Fill pocket & serve.

Nutritional Information (per serving)
CALORIES: 130, TOTAL FAT: 4.5G, SATURATED FAT: 3G, CHOLESTEROL: 15MG, SODIUM: 690MG, CARBOHYDRATES: 7G, FIBER: 0G, SUGAR: 5G, PROTEIN: 14G

Mediterranean Scramble Pocket

Time: 5 minutes
Servings: 1

Ingredients

1 pita half
3 egg whites
2 T chopped tomato
10 spinach leaves, chopped
¼ t oregano
1 T Feta, crumbled

Coat non-stick skillet with cooking spray and place over medium heat. Add all ingredients, stir until set, about 2 minutes. Fill pocket & serve.

Nutritional Information (per serving)

CALORIES: 180, TOTAL FAT: 2.5G, SATURATED FAT: 1.5G, CHOLESTEROL: 10MG, SODIUM: 490MG, CARBOHYDRATES: 22G, FIBER: 7G, SUGAR: 3G, PROTEIN: 18G

Salmon Scramble Pocket

Time: 5 minutes
Servings: 1

Ingredients

1 pita half
3 egg whites
1 slice smoked salmon, chopped (about ½ oz)
1 T reduced fat cream cheese
1 t snipped chives

Coat non-stick skillet with cooking spray and place over medium heat. Add all ingredients, stir until set, about 2 minutes. Fill pocket & serve.

Nutritional Information (per serving)

CALORIES: 170, TOTAL FAT: 2G, SATURATED FAT: 1G, CHOLESTEROL: 10MG, SODIUM: 640MG, CARBOHYDRATES: 18G, FIBER: 4G, SUGAR: 3G, PROTEIN: 18G

entertaining

Pocket Chef Jenna Says...

But what if I have to entertain? Not to worry. Bridal showers, engagement brunches, even cocktail parties are pita friendly. These pitas take buffet table staples and make them Pita Diet friendly.

Crab & Asparagus Pitas

Time: 5 minutes
Servings: 4

Ingredients

    1 (6 oz) can crabmeat
    ½ cup frozen chopped asparagus, thawed
    1 tomato, seeded and chopped
    2 slices provolone cheese, halved
    4 pita halves

In a bowl combine crab, asparagus and tomato. Place one half-slice cheese in each pita. Fill with crab mixture. Warm in microwave, oven, or grill in a pan & serve

Nutritional Information (per serving)

CALORIES: 170, TOTAL FAT: 2.5G, SATURATED FAT: 1.5G, CHOLESTEROL: 50MG, SODIUM: 360MG, CARBOHYDRATES: 19G, FIBER: 5G, SUGAR: 2G, PROTEIN: 16G

 This recipe does not include nutritional information for the pita pocket bread. For this nutritional information, go to page 71.

Broiled Shrimp Pitas

Time: 10 minutes
Servings: 4

Ingredients

    1 cup shrimp
    1 cup reduced fat cheddar cheese
    ¼ cup light mayonnaise
    1 tomato, seeded and chopped
    1 T onion, minced
    2 T parsley, chopped
    4 pita pockets (1/2 each)

In a bowl combine all ingredients. Split one whole pita into two rounds. Spread mixture on each round. Broil 5-6 minutes, or until bubbly and browned & serve.

Nutritional Information (per serving)

CALORIES: 350, TOTAL FAT: 12G, SATURATED FAT: 4.5G, CHOLESTEROL: 190MG, SODIUM: 530MG, CARBOHYDRATES: 21G, FIBER: 4G, SUGAR: 2G, PROTEIN: 36G

This recipe does not include nutritional information for the pita pocket bread. For this nutritional information, go to page 71.

Salami & Olive Pitas

Time: 5 minutes
Servings 2

Ingredients
¼ cup light cream cheese
6 green olives, minced
12 slices reduced-fat salami
2 pita pockets (1/2 each)

In a small bowl combine olives and cream cheese. Spread 2T olive cream cheese in each pita half. Stuff with 6 slices salami & serve.

Nutritional Information (per serving)
CALORIES: 310, TOTAL FAT: 19G, SATURATED FAT: 7G, CHOLESTEROL: 55MG, SODIUM: 1350MG, CARBOHYDRATES: 18G, FIBER: 4G, SUGAR: 2G, PROTEIN: 15G

Cucumber Sandwich Pitas

Time: 5 minutes
Servings 4

Ingredients
1 cucumber, peeled, seeded, thinly sliced
¼ cup light cream cheese
1 T fresh dill, chopped
1 T red horseradish (beets make it red. Use white if you can't find it)
salt & pepper
4 pita pockets (1/2 each)

In a small bowl combine the cream cheese, dill & horseradish. Spread 1 T cheese mixture in each pita. Stuff with cucumber & serve

Nutritional Information (per serving)
Calories: 110, Total Fat: 1.5g, Saturated Fat: 1g, Cholesterol: 5mg, Sodium: 210mg, Carbohydrates: 18g, Fiber: 4g, Sugar: 2g, Protein: 5g

 This recipe does not include nutritional information for the pita pocket bread. For this nutritional information, go to page 71.

Smoked Salmon & Radish Pitas

Time: 5 minutes
Servings: 2

Ingredients

    2 oz smoked salmon, flaked
    ¼ cup light cream cheese
    1 T fresh dill, chopped
    4 radishes, thinly sliced
    salt & pepper
    1 T fresh lemon juice
    2 pita pockets (1/2 each)

In a small bowl combine all ingredients. Fill pitas & serve.

Nutritional Information (per serving)

CALORIES: 160, TOTAL FAT: 4G, SATURATED FAT: 2G, CHOLESTEROL: 15MG, SODIUM: 470MG, CARBOHYDRATES: 18G, FIBER: 4G, SUGAR: 2G, PROTEIN: 11G

Spinach Dip Pitas

Time: 5 minutes
Servings: 4

Ingredients

    1 package frozen chopped spinach, thawed and drained.
    1 t garlic powder
    ½ cup light cream cheese
    ¼ cup light sour cream
    ¼ cup chopped water chestnuts
    1 T fresh lemon juice
    4 pita pockets (1/2 each)

Chop the spinach finely. Combine all ingredients in a bowl. Stuff into pitas & serve.

Nutritional Information (per serving)

CALORIES: 160, TOTAL FAT: 4G, SATURATED FAT: 2.5G, CHOLESTEROL: 15MG, SODIUM: 310MG, CARBOHYDRATES: 23G, FIBER: 6G, SUGAR: 3G, PROTEIN: 9G

 This recipe does not include nutritional information for the pita pocket bread. For this nutritional information, go to page 71.

family style

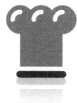

Pocket Chef Jenna Says...

Q: I'm the only one in my family who needs to diet. How would the Pocket Diet work for me.

A: The Pocket Diet will work better for you than other programs because, aside from the pitas used to control your portions, there are no special foods. No counting calories or points, no list of good and bad foods, no metabolic combinations. Just healthy choices and portion control.

You can eat what your family is eating, the only catch is you just get a pita full. The longer you're on the diet the more you'll learn about filling your pita with foods that will keep you feeling full longer, as well as combating cravings by having what you want.

Give it a try with these family style casseroles. Make up the dish, but serve yourself only what fits in a pita. You're family won't even know you're dieting, until the pounds come off.

Breakfast Casserole

Time: 30 minutes
Servings: 6-8

Ingredients
1 bag frozen O'Brien potatoes, thawed (Ore-Ida) (This brand has onions and peppers. If you can't find them add your own)
4 frozen veggie sausage patties, thawed and chopped (Morningstar Farms)
1 bag fat free shredded cheddar (Kraft)
3 eggs
4 egg whites – or 1¼ cups egg substitute in place of eggs & whites
1 can evaporated skim milk
pinch of nutmeg
salt & pepper

Heat oven to 425. Spray a 9x13 casserole dish with cooking spray. In a large bowl mix all ingredients and pour into pan. Bake 20-25 minutes, until golden. Serve in pitas.

Nutritional Information (per serving)
CALORIES: 210, TOTAL FAT: 3.5G, SATURATED FAT: 1G, CHOLESTEROL: 140MG, SODIUM: 950MG, CARBOHYDRATES: 9G, FIBER: 0G, SUGAR: 3G, PROTEIN: 33G

 This recipe does not include nutritional information for the pita pocket bread. For this nutritional information, go to page 71.

Beef Stir Fry

Time: 30 minutes
Servings: 6

Ingredients
12 oz. beef tenderloin or sirloin steak; cut into 1/2" pieces
1 red bell pepper; cut into 1" strips
1 yellow bell pepper
1 cup mushroom (your choice); sliced
1 cup bean sprouts
2 small garlic cloves; crushed
1/2 cup onion; chopped
1 T canola oil
1/4 cup of your favorite beef stir fry marinade (low sodium)

Place beef strips into a small bowl with marinade for at least 10 minutes*. Heat oil in large fry pan on medium heat for 1 minute. Add beef and garlic; stir constantly for 3-4 minutes. Add remaining vegetables. Stir constantly

for 8-10 minutes or until veggies become tender. Add soy sauce to taste
Fill pocket & serve.

The longer the meat sits in the marinade, the more flavor it will absorb.

Nutritional Information (per serving)

CALORIES: 203, TOTAL FAT: 15G,, SATURATED FAT: 5G, CHOLESTEROL: 40MG, SODIUM: 550MG, CARBOHYDRATES: 7G, FIBER: 1G, SUGAR: 1G, PROTEIN: 12G

 This recipe does not include nutritional information for the pita pocket bread. For this nutritional information, go to page 71.

Tex-Mex Egg Casserole

Time: 30 minutes
Servings: 6-8

Ingredients

4 eggs
4 egg whites – or 1½ cups egg substitute in place of eggs & whites
3 cups fat free cottage cheese
1 bag fat free shredded cheddar (Kraft)
1 4 oz can diced green chili
18 reduced fat Ritz crackers, crushed

Heat oven to 350. Spray a 9x13 casserole dish with cooking spray. In a large bowl mix all ingredients except cracker crumbs and pour into pan. Top with cracker crumbs and bake 20-25 minutes, until golden & serve in pitas.

Nutritional Information (per serving)

CALORIES: 420, TOTAL FAT: 28G, SATURATED FAT: 8G, CHOLESTEROL: 115MG, SODIUM: 76MG, CARBOHYDRATES: 26G, FIBER: 2G, SUGAR: 0G, PROTEIN: 16G

 This recipe does not include nutritional information for the pita pocket bread. For this nutritional information, go to page 71.

Hot Chicken Salad

Time: 30 minutes
Servings: 6-8

Ingredients

2½ cups cooked chicken, cubed
1 can slivered water chestnuts, drained (8oz)

1 jar pimentos, drained (8oz)
1 can sliced mushrooms, drained (8oz)
½ cup slivered almonds
2 celery stalks, chopped
1 can reduced fat cream of mushroom soup
2 T lemon juice
1 bag fat free shredded cheddar (Kraft)

Heat oven to 350. Spray a 9x13 casserole dish with cooking spray. Divide cheese in half. In a large bowl mix all ingredients with half of the cheese and pour into pan. Top with remaining cheese and bake 20-25 minutes, until golden & serve in pitas.

Nutritional Information (per serving)

CALORIES: 290, TOTAL FAT: 11G, SATURATED FAT: 2.5G, CHOLESTEROL: 60MG, SODIUM: 770MG, CARBOHYDRATES: 12G, FIBER: 2G, SUGAR: 3G, PROTEIN: 36G

 This recipe does not include nutritional information for the pita pocket bread. For this nutritional information, go to page 71.

Chicken Cacciatore

Time: 30 minutes
Servings: 6-8

Ingredients

1 pound boneless skinless chicken breast, chunked
1 can Italian stewed tomatoes
1 zucchini, chopped
1 bell pepper, chopped
½ onion, chopped
1 T Italian seasoning
1 can tomato sauce (8 oz)
1 T bottled minced garlic.

Heat oven to 425. Spray a 9x13 casserole dish with cooking spray. In a large bowl mix all ingredients and pour into pan. Bake 20-25 minutes, until chicken is cooked through and sauce has thickened & serve.

Nutritional Information (per serving)

CALORIES: 180, TOTAL FAT: 3G, SATURATED FAT: 1G, CHOLESTEROL: 65MG, SODIUM: 480MG, CARBOHYDRATES: 12G, FIBER: 2G, SUGAR: 6G, PROTEIN: 25G

Tip: Serve in a pita sprinkled with parmesan. Your family may like it over pasta.

 This recipe does not include nutritional information for the pita pocket bread. For this nutritional information, go to page 71.

fish stick
pockets

Pocket Chef Jenna Says...

Use your favorite brand of fish sticks to create these tasty pita sandwiches. Frozen breaded fish fillets work great here as well. Prepare them according to the package directions, and then assemble the pitas.

Fish Stick Club Pita

Time: 5 minutes
Servings: 1

Ingredients

1 pita half
2-3 Fish Sticks
1 slice cooked bacon
1 leaf lettuce
2 slices tomato
1 T mayo

Spread mayo inside pita pocket. Fill with other ingredients & serve.

Nutritional Information (per serving)

CALORIES: 420, TOTAL FAT: 28G, SATURATED FAT: 8G, CHOLESTEROL: 115MG, SODIUM: 76MG, CARBOHYDRATES: 26G, FIBER: 2G, SUGAR: 0G, PROTEIN: 16G

Honey Mustard Fish Stick Pita

Time: 5 minutes (once fish is ready)
Servings: 1

Ingredients

1 pita half
2-3 Fish Sticks
1 leaf lettuce
2 slices tomato
1 slice reduced-fat cheddar
1 T honey mustard

Spread honey mustard inside pita. Fill with other ingredients & serve.

Nutritional Information (per serving)

CALORIES: 370, TOTAL FAT: 18G, SATURATED FAT: 7G, CHOLESTEROL: 110MG, SODIUM: 760MG, CARBOHYDRATES: 29G, FIBER: 05G, SUGAR: 9G, PROTEIN: 22G

Fish Stick Parmesan

Time: 5 minutes (once fish is ready)
Servings: 1

Ingredients
  1 pita half
  2-3 Fish Sticks
  2 T marinara
  1 T parmesan

Spread marinara inside pita. Fill wish fish sticks and sprinkle with Parmesan & serve.

Nutritional Information (per serving)
CALORIES: 280, TOTAL FAT: 13G, SATURATED FAT: 4G, CHOLESTEROL: 100MG, SODIUM: 770MG, CARBOHYDRATES: 24G, FIBER: 0G, SUGAR: 3G, PROTEIN: 16G

Ranch Fish Stick Pita

Time: 5 minutes (once fish is ready)
Servings: 1

Ingredients
  1 pita half
  2-3 Fish Sticks
  1 leaf lettuce
  2 slices tomato
  1 T light ranch
  1 t red onion, minced

Spread ranch inside pita pocket. Fill with remaining ingredients & serve.

Nutritional Information (per serving)
CALORIES: 260, TOTAL FAT: 10G, SATURATED FAT: 10G, CHOLESTEROL: 95MG, SODIUM: 650MG, CARBOHYDRATES: 28G, FIBER: 0G, SUGAR: 4G, PROTEIN: 14G

Fish Tacos

Time: 5 minutes (once fish is ready)
Servings: 1

Ingredients
1 pita half
2-3 Fish Sticks
1 T fat-free plain yogurt
1 T Salsa
¼ cup shredded cabbage

In a small bowl combine salsa & yogurt. Spread inside pita. Fill with fish sticks and cabbage & serve.

Nutritional Information (per serving)
CALORIES: 250, TOTAL FAT: 11G, SATURATED FAT: 3G, CHOLESTEROL: 95MG, SODIUM: 610MG, CARBOHYDRATES: 24G, FIBER: 0G, SUGAR: 4G, PROTEIN: 14G

Fish Stick Melt

Time: 5 minutes (once fish is ready)
Servings: 1

Ingredients
1 pita half
2-3 Fish Sticks
1 Tomato slice
1 slice reduced-fat American cheese

Arrange ingredients inside pita. Grill in nonstick pan coated with cooking spray over medium heat 1 minute on each side or until cheese is melted & serve.

Nutritional Information (per serving)
CALORIES: 240, TOTAL FAT: 11G, SATURATED FAT: 3G, CHOLESTEROL: 95MG, SODIUM: 540MG, CARBOHYDRATES: 21G, FIBER: 0G, SUGAR: 2G, PROTEIN: 14G

BBQ Fish Stick Pita

Time: 5 minutes (once fish is ready)
Servings: 1

Ingredients

1 pita half
2-3 Fish Sticks
1 grilled onion slice
1 T BBQ sauce
1 leaf lettuce
2 slices tomato

Coat a non-stick pan with cooking spray. Place over medium-high heat. Grill one onion slice until it begins to brown. Spread BBQ sauce inside pita. Stuff with grilled onion & remaining ingredients & serve.

Nutritional Information (per serving)

Calories: 280, Total Fat: 10g, Saturated Fat: 2.5g, Cholesterol: 95mg, Sodium: 710mg, Carbohydrates: 21g, Fiber: 1g, Sugar: 10g, Protein: 14g

fruit pockets

Pita Pop Tart

Time: 5 minutes
Servings: 1

Ingredients
　 1 pita half
　 1 T jam or preserves

Spread preserves inside pita. Toast in toaster oven or grill in non-stick pan coated with cooking spray & serve.

Nutritional Information (per serving)
CALORIES: 130, TOTAL FAT: 0G, SATURATED FAT: 0G, CHOLESTEROL: 0MG, SODIUM: 150MG, CARBOHYDRATES: 29G, FIBER: 4G, SUGAR: 8G, PROTEIN: 3G

Pita Danish

Time: 5 minutes
Servings: 1

Ingredients
　 1 pita half
　 1 T cheesecake cream cheese
　 1 T jam or preserves

Spread cream cheese and preserves inside pita. Warm in microwave for 30 seconds & serve.

Nutritional Information (per serving)
CALORIES: 180, TOTAL FAT: 3G, SATURATED FAT: 3G, CHOLESTEROL: 15MG, SODIUM: 190MG, CARBOHYDRATES: 29G, FIBER: 4G, SUGAR: 11G, PROTEIN: 4G

Pineapple Pitas

Time: 5 minutes
Servings: 4

Ingredients
   4 pita half
   1 cup fat free cream cheese, softened
   1 can crushed pineapple (4 oz), drained
   2 T dry roasted peanuts, chopped

In a small bowl combine all ingredients. Spread inside pitas & enjoy.

Nutritional Information (per serving)
CALORIES: 170, TOTAL FAT: 2.5G, SATURATED FAT: 0G, CHOLESTEROL: 5MG, SODIUM: 450MG, CARBOHYDRATES: 24G, FIBER: 5G, SUGAR: 6G, PROTEIN: 13G

Peanut Fruit Salad

Time: 5 minutes
Servings: 4

Ingredients
   4 pita halves
   1 T creamy peanut butter
   3 T vanilla yogurt
   1 ½ cup sliced strawberries
   2 bananas, sliced
   1 small can mandarin oranges, drained
   1 T dry roasted peanuts, chopped

In a small bowl combine peanut butter and yogurt. Stir with fruit and peanuts. Fill pitas & serve.

Nutritional Information (per serving)
CALORIES: 200, TOTAL FAT: 3G, SATURATED FAT: .5G, CHOLESTEROL: 0MG, SODIUM: 180MG, CARBOHYDRATES: 40G, FIBER: 7G, SUGAR: 19G, PROTEIN: 6G

Date & Walnut Spread

Time: 5 minutes
Servings: 4

Ingredients
4 oz. whipped cream cheese; low fat
1/3 cup pitted dates; chopped
1/4 cup walnuts; chopped
1 tsp. cinnamon

Mix the dates, walnuts and cream cheese. Sprinkle with cinnamon. Spread 2 tablespoons into pocket & serve.

Nutritional Information (per serving)
CALORIES: 155, TOTAL FAT: 9G, SATURATED FAT: 3G, CHOLESTEROL: 16MG, SODIUM: 84MG, CARBOHYDRATES: 14G, FIBER: 2G, SUGAR: 9G, PROTEIN: 5G

 This recipe does not include nutritional information for the pita pocket bread. For this nutritional information, go to page 71.

Crunchy Key Lime Banana

Time: 5 minutes
Servings: 2

Ingredients
1/2 banana; sliced
3 T key lime pie yogurt; fat free (no sugar added)
T crunchy wheat & barley cereal or granola

Mix yogurt with banana and cereal. Fill pocket & serve.

Nutritional Information (per serving)
CALORIES: 86, TOTAL FAT: TRACE, SATURATED FAT: TRACE, CHOLESTEROL: 1MG, SODIUM: 40MG, CARBOHYDRATES: 1G, FIBER: 2G, SUGAR: 10G, PROTEIN: 3G

 This recipe does not include nutritional information for the pita pocket bread. For this nutritional information, go to page 71.

Creamy Summer Berry Pocket

Time: 3 minutes
Servings: 1

Ingredients

    1/2 cup fresh berries (raspberry, strawberry, blueberry or blackberry)
    1 T whipped cream cheese; low fat
    1 T sugar-free preserves (use a matching berry preserve)

Spread inside of pocket with cream cheese. Spread the other inside pocket with the preserve. Add the berries & serve.

Nutritional Information (per serving)

CALORIES: 82, TOTAL FAT: 3G, SATURATED FAT: 1G, CHOLESTEROL: 8MG, SODIUM: 45MG, CARBOHYDRATES: 13G, FIBER: 2G, SUGAR: 10G, PROTEIN: 2G

 This recipe does not include nutritional information for the pita pocket bread. For this nutritional information, go to page 71.

fruit salad
pockets

Strawberry Parmesan Salad

Time 5 minutes
Servings: 2

Ingredients

 1 cup romaine, shredded
 ¼ cup strawberries, sliced
 1 T red onion, diced
 1 T slivered almonds
 1 T parmesan cheese, grated
 1 T honey
 1 T balsamic vinegar

In a small bowl combine honey and vinegar. Toss in remaining ingredients. Fill pita & serve.

Nutritional Information (per serving)

CALORIES: 60, TOTAL FAT: 2G, SATURATED FAT: .5MG, CHOLESTEROL: 0MG, SODIUM: 40MG, CARBOHYDRATES: 10G, FIBER: 3, SUGAR: 8G, PROTEIN: 2G

 This recipe does not include nutritional information for the pita pocket bread. For this nutritional information, go to page 71.

Honey Vanilla Fruit Salad

Time 5 minutes
Servings: 2

Ingredients

 2 T light vanilla yogurt
 1 T light mayonnaise
 1 ½ t honey
 pinch ground giner
 pinch cinnamon
 1 Red Delicious apple, cubed
 1 ripe pear, cubed
 1 orange, sectioned
 2 T raisins

Mix first five ingredients until smooth. Stir in fruits. Fill pita & serve.

Nutritional Information (per serving)
CALORIES: 130, TOTAL FAT: 2G, SATURATED FAT: 0MG, CHOLESTEROL: 0MG, SODIUM: 40MG, CARBOHYDRATES: 31G, FIBER: 4, SUGAR: 24G, PROTEIN: 1G

 This recipe does not include nutritional information for the pita pocket bread. For this nutritional information, go to page 71.

Creamy Citrus Fruit Salad

Time 5 minutes
Servings: 2

Ingredients
1 small can mandarin oranges, drained
1 small can pineapple tidbits, drained
1 small orange, peeled and chopped
2 T light vanilla yogurt
1 t frozen orange juice concentrate
1 T flaked coconut

In a small bowl combine all ingredients. Fill pita & serve.

Nutritional Information (per serving)
CALORIES: 160, TOTAL FAT: 4G, SATURATED FAT: 2.5MG, CHOLESTEROL: 10MG, SODIUM: 115MG, CARBOHYDRATES: 25G, FIBER: 3, SUGAR: 20G, PROTEIN: 7G

 This recipe does not include nutritional information for the pita pocket bread. For this nutritional information, go to page 71.

Cheesy Fruit Salad

Time 5 minutes
Servings: 2

Ingredients
1 apple, diced
1 pear, diced
1 ounce reduced fat cheddar, diced
1 ounce reduced fat Monterey jack, diced
½ cup seedless grapes, halved
3 T light raspberry yogurt

In a small bowl combine all ingredients. Fill pita & serve.

Nutritional Information (per serving)

CALORIES: 100, TOTAL FAT: 1G, SATURATED FAT: .0MG, CHOLESTEROL: 0MG, SODIUM: 0MG, CARBOHYDRATES: 25G, FIBER: 3G, SUGAR: 21G, PROTEIN: 2G

 This recipe does not include nutritional information for the pita pocket bread. For this nutritional information, go to page 71.

Ham & Pineapple Salad Pitas

Time 5 minutes
Servings: 4

Ingredients

1 cup cooked ham, diced
½ cup celery, chopped
¼ cup green pepper, chopped
¼ cup light mayonnaise
½ t mustard
1 small can pineapple tidbits, drained and chopped

In a small bowl combine all ingredients. Fill pita & serve.

Nutritional Information (per serving)

CALORIES: 100, TOTAL FAT: 7G, SATURATED FAT: 2.5MG, CHOLESTEROL: 30MG, SODIUM: 105MG, CARBOHYDRATES: 3G, FIBER: 2G, SUGAR: 2G, PROTEIN: 8G

 This recipe does not include nutritional information for the pita pocket bread. For this nutritional information, go to page 71.

grilled cheese
pockets

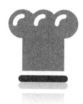

Pocket Chef Jenna Says...

Grilled Cheese isn't just for kiddos anymore. Adults are rediscovering the tasty treat and giving it a new name – panini. A panini is a grilled sandwich made on a press.

Because pita pockets hold fillings together, you can grill the sandwiches normally in a pan (1 minute each side), buy a panini press, use your George Foreman Grill, or even your waffle iron! Whatever option suits you, be sure to use a spritz of cooking spray to stay out of sticky situations.

Can't lug the panini grill to work or school? No problem. These are all great as they are, or microwaved for 20-30 seconds.

The Classic Grilled Cheese Pocket

Time: 5 minutes
Servings: 1

Ingredients
1 slice Reduced-fat American cheese
1/2 Pita Pocket

Place in pita, grill & serve.

Nutritional Information (per serving)
CALORIES: 130, TOTAL FAT: 1G, SATURATED FAT: 0G, CHOLESTEROL: 5MG, SODIUM: 310MG, CARBOHYDRATES: 17G, FIBER: 4G, SUGAR: 1G, PROTEIN: 10G

The Traditional Grilled Cheese Pocket

Time: 5 minutes
Servings: 1

Ingredients
1 slice Reduced Fat Cheddar
1 Tomato slice
1/2 Pita Pocket

Place in pita, grill & serve.

Nutritional Information (per serving)
CALORIES: 130, TOTAL FAT: 2G, SATURATED FAT: 1G, CHOLESTEROL: 5MG, SODIUM: 320MG, CARBOHYDRATES: 17G, FIBER: 4G, SUGAR: 2G, PROTEIN: 10G

Ham & Swiss Grilled Cheese Pocket

Time: 5 minutes
Servings: 1

Ingredients
2 slices Ham lunchmeat
1 slice reduced-fat Swiss
1/2 Pita Pocket

Place in pita, grill & serve

Nutritional Information (per serving)
CALORIES: 300, TOTAL FAT: 11G, SATURATED FAT: 6G, CHOLESTEROL: 45MG,
SODIUM: 1380MG, CARBOHYDRATES: 25G, FIBER: 4G, SUGAR: 6G, PROTEIN: 26G

Bacon, Cheese & Tomato Pocket

Time: 5 minutes
Servings: 1

Ingredients

2 oz. cheddar cheese; low fat (monterey jack, provolone, or swiss)
2 oz. canadian bacon or ham
2 tomato slices
1/2 Pita Pocket

Heat meat in microwave for 10 seconds on high. Layer cheese, tomato and meat in pocket. Toast the filled pocket on med-high & serve.

Nutritional Information (per serving)

CALORIES: 176, TOTAL FAT: 7G, SATURATED FAT: 3G, CHOLESTEROL: 42MG,
SODIUM*: 500MG, CARBOHYDRATES: 4G, FIBER: TRACE, SUGAR: 2G, PROTEIN: 24G

Turkey, Apple Grilled Cheese Pocket

Time: 5 minutes
Servings: 1

Ingredients

2 slices Smoked Turkey lunchmeat
¼ Apple, sliced thin
1 slice Reduced-fat cheddar
1/2 Pita Pocket

Place in pita, grill & serve

Nutritional Information (per serving)

CALORIES: 180, TOTAL FAT: 6G, SATURATED FAT: 1.5G, CHOLESTEROL: 10MG,
SODIUM: 590MG, CARBOHYDRATES: 23G, FIBER: 4G, SUGAR: 3G, PROTEIN: 8G

Grilled Blue Cheese with Apricots Pocket

Time: 5 minutes
Servings: 1

Ingredients
    2 slices Roasted turkey lunchmeat
    1 t Blue cheese, crumbled
    1 T light Mayonnaise
    1 T Sugar free apricot preserves
    2 spinach leaves
    1/2 Pita Pocket

In a small bowl combine mayonnaise and blue cheese. Spread inside half of pita. Spread preserves on other half. Stuff with turkey and spinach. Grill & serve.

Nutritional Information (per serving)
CALORIES: 180, TOTAL FAT: 6G, SATURATED FAT: 1.5G, CHOLESTEROL: 10MG, SODIUM: 590MG, CARBOHYDRATES: 23G, FIBER: 4G, SUGAR: 3G, PROTEIN: 8G

Spicy Grilled Cheese Pocket

Time: 5 minutes
Servings: 1

Ingredients
    1 slice Reduced fat pepper jack
    2 slices Roasted turkey lunchmeat
    1 Roasted red pepper (bottled)
    1/2 Pita Pocket

Place in pita, grill & serve.

Nutritional Information (per serving)
CALORIES: 160, TOTAL FAT: 5G, SATURATED FAT: 2.5G, CHOLESTEROL: 25MG, SODIUM: 540MG, CARBOHYDRATES: 17G, FIBER: 4G, SUGAR: 1G, PROTEIN: 11G

Cuban Grilled Cheese Pocket

Time: 5 minutes
Servings: 1

Ingredients

    1 T Dijon mustard
    2 slices Ham lunchmeat
    1 slice reduced-fat Swiss
    1 dill pickle, sandwich slices (long vertical slice)
    3 peppercini rings
    1/2 Pita Pocket

Spread mustard inside pita. Stuff with remaining ingredients. Grill & serve.

Nutritional Information (per serving)

CALORIES: 250, TOTAL FAT: 8G, SATURATED FAT: 4G, CHOLESTEROL: 45MG, SODIUM: 2470MG, CARBOHYDRATES: 20G, FIBER: 5G, SUGAR: 3G, PROTEIN: 19G

Panini Grilled Cheese

Time: 5 minutes
Servings: 1

Ingredients

    1 slice Prosciutto
    1 Roasted Red pepper (bottled)
    ¼ cup reduced fat mozzarella, shredded
    1/2 Pita Pocket

Place in pita, grill & serve.

Nutritional Information (per serving)

CALORIES: 220, TOTAL FAT: 7G, SATURATED FAT: 4G, CHOLESTEROL: 30MG, SODIUM: 770MG, CARBOHYDRATES: 20G, FIBER: 4G, SUGAR: 4G, PROTEIN: 15G

Vegetarian Panini

Time: 5 minutes
Servings: 1

Ingredients
1 Roasted Red pepper (bottled)
¼ cup reduced fat mozzarella, shredded
1 sundried tomato, chopped
1 T reduced fat pesto
1/2 Pita Pocket

Spread pesto inside pita. Stuff with remaining ingredients, grill & serve.

Nutritional Information (per serving)
CALORIES: 220, TOTAL FAT: 7G, SATURATED FAT: 3.5G, CHOLESTEROL: 20MG, SODIUM: 430MG, CARBOHYDRATES: 23G, FIBER: 5G, SUGAR: 5G, PROTEIN: 12G

Turkey Panini

Time: 5 minutes
Servings: 1

Ingredients
1 t light mayonnaise
1 t reduced fat pesto
2 slices turkey lunchmeat
1 roasted red pepper (bottled)
½ slice provolone
1/2 Pita Pocket

In a small bowl combine mayonnaise & pesto. Spread inside pita. Stuff with remaining ingredients, grill & serve.

Nutritional Information (per serving)
CALORIES: 290, TOTAL FAT: 13G, SATURATED FAT: 6G, CHOLESTEROL: 40MG, SODIUM: 1180MG, CARBOHYDRATES: 20G, FIBER: 4G, SUGAR: 3G, PROTEIN: 20G

Grilled Blue Cheese Pockets

Time: 10 minutes
Servings: 4

Ingredients
4 pita halves
¼ cup crumbled blue cheese
¼ cup light cream cheese
8 tomato slices
16 basil leaves

In a small bowl combine cheeses. Spread inside pitas. Arrange tomato and basil inside. Grill & serve.

Nutritional Information (per serving)
Calories: 150, Total Fat: 5g, Saturated Fat: 3.5g, Cholesterol: 15mg, Sodium: 300mg, Carbohydrates: 18g, Fiber: 4g, Sugar: 3g, Protein: 7g

grilling greats

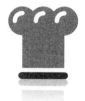

Pocket Chef Jenna Says...

When barbeque season hits, bring along a bag of pitas. I would set them next to the hot dog and hamburger buns. It got people interested in the program, and they tried it as well. You can thank my neighbor for the hot dog potato salad combo.

Hot Dog Pockets

Time: 5 minutes
Servings 1

Ingredients
    1 pita half
    1 hot dog, cooked and sliced
    Ketchup (or mustard)

Slice grilled hotdog and arrange in pita. Squirt on your favorite condiment & serve.

Nutritional Information (per serving)
CALORIES: 240, TOTAL FAT: 20G, SATURATED FAT: 8G, CHOLESTEROL: 40MG, SODIUM: 670MG, CARBOHYDRATES: 6G, FIBER: 2G, SUGAR: 1G, PROTEIN: 11G

Hot Dog Pocket Deluxe

Time: 5 minutes
Servings 1

Ingredients
    1 pita half
    1 hot dog, cooked and sliced
    2 T sauerkraut
    1 t onion, minced
    1 t mustard

Fill pita with hot dog slices. Top with sauerkraut, onions, mustard & serve.

Nutritional Information (per serving)
CALORIES: 270, TOTAL FAT: 17G, SATURATED FAT: 7G, CHOLESTEROL: 35MG, SODIUM: 860MG, CARBOHYDRATES: 19G, FIBER: 5G, SUGAR: 3G, PROTEIN: 10G

Hot Dog & Potato Salad Pita

Time: 5 minutes
Servings 1
Ingredients
    1 pita half
    1 hot dog, cooked and sliced
    ¼ cup potato salad
    2 tomato slices

Arrange hot dog, salad & tomato in pita & serve.

Nutritional Information (per serving)
CALORIES: 360, TOTAL FAT: 22G, SATURATED FAT: 8G, CHOLESTEROL: 75MG, SODIUM: 1060MG, CARBOHYDRATES: 26G, FIBER: 5G, SUGAR: 5G, PROTEIN: 12G

Sausage & Pepper Pitas

Time: 5 minutes
Servings 2

Ingredients
    2 pita halves
    1 Italian sausage, grilled and sliced (3 oz)
    ½ green pepper, sliced
    ½ onion, sliced
    1 slice provolone cheese, halved

While sausage is grilling sauté pepper and onion in a non-stick pan coated with cooking spray until softened, about 3 minutes. Arrange sausage slices and cheese in each pita. Top with vegetable mixture & serve.

Nutritional Information (per serving)
CALORIES: 200, TOTAL FAT: 9G, SATURATED FAT: 3G, CHOLESTEROL: 25MG, SODIUM: 450MG, CARBOHYDRATES: 19G, FIBER: 5G, SUGAR: 3G, PROTEIN: 10G

hummus

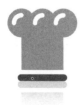

Pocket Chef Jenna Says...

There is nothing more perfect for a pita than hummus. Grab a tub from your grocer's deli section, or mix up one of these tantalizing options.

Hummus Pita

Time: 5 minutes
Servings: 1

Ingredients
    1 pita half
    ¼ cup prepared hummus
    1 lettuce leaf
    2 cucumber slices
    2 tomato slices
    1 onion slice

Spread hummus inside pita. Fill with lettuce cucumber & tomato & serve.

Nutritional Information (per serving)
CALORIES: 200, TOTAL FAT: 5G, SATURATED FAT: 1G, CHOLESTEROL: 0MG, SODIUM: 290MG, CARBOHYDRATES: 32G, FIBER: 8G, SUGAR: 4G, PROTEIN: 7G

Roasted Red Pepper Hummus

Time: 5 minutes
Servings: 4

Ingredients
    1 cup bottled roasted red peppers
    1 can (15 oz) garbanzo beans, drained
    2 T bottled minced garlic
    1 T extra virgin olive oil
    juice of one lemon
    1 t oregano
    salt & pepper
    4 pita halves

Place all ingredients in a food processor and puree. Spoon into pita pockets & serve.

Nutritional Information (per serving)
CALORIES: 250, TOTAL FAT: 6G, SATURATED FAT: .5G, CHOLESTEROL: 0MG, SODIUM: 580MG, CARBOHYDRATES: 40G, FIBER: 10G, SUGAR: 3G, PROTEIN: 9G

Toasted Sesame Hummus

Time: 5 minutes
Servings: 4

Ingredients

1 can (15 oz) garbanzo beans, drained
2 T bottled minced garlic
1 T extra virgin olive oil
1 T toasted sesame oil
juice of one lemon
salt & pepper
4 pita halves

Place all ingredients in a food processor and puree. Spoon into pita pockets & serve.

Nutritional Information (per serving)

Calories: 260, Total Fat: 9g, Saturated Fat: 1g, Cholesterol: 0mg, Sodium: 370mg, Carbohydrates: 37g, Fiber: 10g, Sugar: 2g, Protein: 8g

international

Spring Roll Pockets

Time: 15 minutes
Servings: 5

Ingredients

1 egg
2 egg whites
2 green onions, chopped
1 cup bean sprouts
5 lettuce leaves
5 krab legs
½ t sesame oil
¼ cup bottled sweet chili sauce

In a small bowl beat eggs until combined. Place a non-stick pan over medium heat and spray with cooking spray. Add eggs and cook into a round (like a pancake). Remove from pan & let cool before slicing into strips. In a bowl combine green onions and sprouts. Sprinkle sesame oil over Krab legs. Line each pita with lettuce. Add krab leg, egg strips, and sprout mixture. Drizzle sweet chili sauce over the top, or use for dipping & serve.

Nutritional Information (per serving)

CALORIES: 100, TOTAL FAT: 2G, SATURATED FAT: 0G, CHOLESTEROL: 65MG, SODIUM: 420MG, CARBOHYDRATES: 11G, FIBER: 0G, SUGAR: 1G, PROTEIN: 10G

 This recipe does not include nutritional information for the pita pocket bread. For this nutritional information, go to page 71.

Indian Samosa

Time: 20 minutes
Servings: 4

Ingredients

½ pound ground lamb
4 green onions, chopped
2 t curry paste
4 dried apricots, chopped
1 potato, diced
2 t apricot chutney
4 T frozen peas
¼ cup hot water
1 T cilantro, chopped

In a small lidded saucepan brown ground lamb. Add onions, curry, apricots, potato, chutney, and water. Cover and simmer 10 minutes, until potato is tender. Stir in peas and cilantro. Fill pitas & serve. If desired, serve with Raita (Page 183).

Nutritional Information (per serving)
CALORIES: 300, TOTAL FAT: 17G, SATURATED FAT: 8G, CHOLESTEROL: 55MG, SODIUM: 180MG, CARBOHYDRATES: 23G, FIBER: 3G, SUGAR: 13G, PROTEIN: 14G

 This recipe does not include nutritional information for the pita pocket bread. For this nutritional information, go to page 71.

Thai Beef Salad

Time: 10 minutes
Servings: 4-6

Ingredients
½ pound thinly sliced grilled steak
1 cup shredded leaf lettuce
1 tomato, seeded and chopped
2 green onions, sliced
½ cucumber, peeled, seeded, sliced
4 mint leaves, thinly sliced
1 T cilantro, chopped
1 T bottled minced garlic
1 small red chili pepper, seeded, minced
2 T fish sauce
3 T lime juice
1 T rice vinegar

Combine all ingredients in a small bowl. Stuff into pitas and serve.

Nutritional Information (per serving)
CALORIES: 120, TOTAL FAT: 4G, SATURATED FAT: 1.5G, CHOLESTEROL: 40MG, SODIUM: 760MG, CARBOHYDRATES: 6G, FIBER: 1G, SUGAR: 2G, PROTEIN: 15G

 This recipe does not include nutritional information for the pita pocket bread. For this nutritional information, go to page 71.

italian
pockets

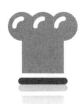

Pocket Chef Jenna Says...

Let no craving go unsatisfied. These options are a treat for the tongue, and much faster to prepare than their traditional versions.

Meatball Pita

Time: 5 minutes
Serves: 1

Ingredients

3 frozen meatballs, cooked
2 T prepared marinara
2 T low fat mozzarella
1 T Parmesan
2 Pita pockets (1/2 each)

In a small bowl combine meatballs and marinara. Spoon meatballs into pitas. Top with cheese & serve.

Nutritional Information (per serving)

CALORIES: 350, TOTAL FAT: 16G, SATURATED FAT: 7G, CHOLESTEROL: 80MG, SODIUM: 850MG, CARBOHYDRATES: 25G, FIBER: 4G, SUGAR: 1G, PROTEIN: 24G

Italian Sandwich Pita

Time: 5 minutes
Serves 1

Ingredients

1 pita half
2 t light mayo
1 t light Italian dressing
3 slices Italian meats
    (salami, ham, pepperoni, mortadella – your choice)
½ slice Provolone cheese
1 lettuce leaf
2 tomato slices
2 green pepper strips
1 onion slice

Combine mayo and dressing. Spread inside pita. Arrange meat and cheese inside. Fill with vegetables & serve.

Nutritional Information (per serving)

CALORIES: 280, TOTAL FAT: 15G, SATURATED FAT: 6G, CHOLESTEROL: 35MG, SODIUM: 730MG, CARBOHYDRATES: 23G, FIBER: 5G, SUGAR: 5G, PROTEIN: 15G

Panzanella in a Pocket

Time: 10 minutes
Serves: 2

Ingredients

 3 tomatoes, seeded & chopped
 ¼ red onion, thinly sliced
 2 T Parmesan, shredded
 ½ bell pepper, chopped
 1 T mint, chopped
 1 T basil, chopped
 1 T parsley, chopped
 I T extra virgin olive oil
 1 T red wine vinegar
 salt & pepper
 2 Pita pockets (1/2 each)

Mix all ingredients in a bowl. Spoon into pitas & serve.

Nutritional Information (per serving)

CALORIES: 240, TOTAL FAT: 10G, SATURATED FAT: 2G, CHOLESTEROL: 5MG, SODIUM: 270MG, CARBOHYDRATES: 29G, FIBER: 6G, SUGAR: 9G, PROTEIN: 8G

Antipasto Pitas

Time: 5 minutes
Serves: 4

Ingredients

 4 slices reduced fat salami
 1 cup jarred giardiniera vegetables, drained and chopped
 1/4 cup jarred roasted red pepper, drained and chopped
 2 T cup peperoncini rings
 4 slices reduced fat mozzarella
 1 cup arugula or spinach leaves
 4 Pita pockets (1/2 each)

In a bowl toss vegetables together. Line pitas with cheese, salami and arugula. Stuff with vegetable salad & serve.

CALORIES: 210, TOTAL FAT: 6G, SATURATED FAT: 2G, CHOLESTEROL: 20MG, SODIUM: 950MG, CARBOHYDRATES: 26G, FIBER: 5G, SUGAR: 3G, PROTEIN: 11G

Zucchini Parmesan Pockets

Time: 30 minutes
Serves: 4-6

Ingredients
1 zucchini, thinly sliced
2 T milk
¼ cup cracker meal or crushed crackers
¼ cup parmesan
1 T spaghetti sauce seasoning
½ cup prepared marinara
3 slices Provolone cheese, halved
6 Pita pockets (1/2 each)

Heat oven to 400. Place a rack on top of a cookie sheet. Spritz with cooking spray. Pour milk into a plate. On another plate combine cracker meal, parmesan, and spices. Dip each zucchini slice in milk, dredge in crumb mixture, and place on rack. Repeat with remaining zucchini slices. Bake 20 minutes, until brown and crispy. Spread inside of pitas with sauce. Arrange cheese and zucchini slices inside & serve.

Nutritional Information (per serving)
CALORIES: 170, TOTAL FAT: 5G, SATURATED FAT: 2.5G, CHOLESTEROL: 10MG, SODIUM: 370MG, CARBOHYDRATES: 24G, FIBER: 5G, SUGAR: 3G, PROTEIN: 8G

Roasted Portobello Pita

Time: 20 minutes
Serves: 2

Ingredients
2 portobello mushrooms, cleaned and halved
4 thick slices red onion
1 red pepper, cut into strips
¼ cup light Balsamic vinaigrette
¼ cup light mayonnaise
¼ cup Parmesan
2 Pita pockets (1/2 each)

In a small bowl toss vegetables with vinaigrette. Heat oven to 450. Place vegetables on a cookie sheet. Roast for 10 minutes, turn, then roast 5 minutes more. Spread mayo inside pitas. Sprinkle with Parmesan. Fill with roasted vegetables & serve.

Nutritional Information (per serving)
CALORIES: 300, TOTAL FAT: 14G, SATURATED FAT: 3.5G, CHOLESTEROL: 20MG, SODIUM: 600MG, CARBOHYDRATES: 34G, FIBER: 8G, SUGAR: 12G, PROTEIN: 11G

Caprese Pita

Time: 5 minutes
Serves 1

Ingredients
    1 pita half
    2 slices fresh tomato
    1 slice fresh mozzarella
    2 basil leaves
    1 t extra virgin olive oil

Stuff pita & serve.

Nutritional Information (per serving)
CALORIES: 210, TOTAL FAT: 10G, SATURATED FAT: 4G, CHOLESTEROL: 15MG, SODIUM: 310MG, CARBOHYDRATES: 19G, FIBER: 4G, SUGAR: 2G, PROTEIN: 11G

Goat Cheese and Red Pepper

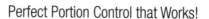

Time: 5 minutes
Serves 1

Ingredients
    1 pita half
    2 T goat cheese
    2 T bottled roasted red pepper
    6 arugula leaves
Stuff pita & serve.

Nutritional Information (per serving)
CALORIES: 190, TOTAL FAT: 9G, SATURATED FAT: 6G, CHOLESTEROL: 20MG, SODIUM: 340MG, CARBOHYDRATES: 18G, FIBER: 4G, SUGAR: 2G, PROTEIN: 10G

kabobs

Pocket Chef Jenna Says...

You want to talk portion control? Kabobs are another secret, useful for dining out. Usually, what fits on an 8 inch skewer fits in a pita. Kabobs are also great when not everyone in your family is dieting. They'll never know you're sneaking in your 'diet' food into their regular meal times.

Kabob Tip! Be careful of the handles on metal skewers. They can get very hot. If using bamboo skewers be sure to soak in water for at least 30 minutes to keep them from burning.

Souvlaki w/ Tzatziki

Time: 15 minutes
Servings: 4-8 skewers

Ingredients

> 1 zucchini, quartered and chunked
> ½ pounds boneless skinless chicken breasts, cut into 1 inch pieces
> juice of one lemon
> 1 T extra virgin olive oil
> salt & pepper
> 2 garlic cloves, crushed

In a small bowl combine lemon juice, olive oil, garlic, salt and pepper. Marinade chicken for at least 5-30 minutes. Thread onto skewers, alternating with zucchini chunks. Grill 8 minutes. Pull from the skewer and stuff into pita. Serve with Tzatziki.

Nutritional Information (per serving)

CALORIES: 120, TOTAL FAT: 1G, SATURATED FAT: 0G, CHOLESTEROL: 0MG, SODIUM: 175MG, CARBOHYDRATES: 14G, FIBER: 8G, SUGAR: 2G, PROTEIN: 8G

 This recipe does not include nutritional information for the pita pocket bread. For this nutritional information, go to page 71.

Tzatziki

Time: 5 minutes
Servings: 4

Ingredients

> 1 cucumber, peeled, seeded, grated
> ½ cup plain non-fat yogurt
> salt & pepper
> 1 T lemon juice
> 1 t crushed garlic

Combine all ingredients in a small bowl.

Nutritional Information (per serving)

CALORIES: 120, TOTAL FAT: 1G, SATURATED FAT: 0G, CHOLESTEROL: 0MG, SODIUM: 175MG, CARBOHYDRATES: 14G, FIBER: 8G, SUGAR: 2G, PROTEIN: 8G

This recipe does not include nutritional information for the pita pocket bread. For this nutritional information, go to page 71.

Raita

Time: 5 minutes
Servings: 4

Ingredients

1 cucumber, peeled, seeded, grated
½ cup plain non-fat yogurt
salt & pepper
2 chopped green onion
1 t crushed garlic

Combine all ingredients in a small bowl.

Nutritional Information (per serving)

CALORIES: 120, TOTAL FAT: 1G, SATURATED FAT: 0G, CHOLESTEROL: 0MG, SODIUM: 175MG, CARBOHYDRATES: 14G, FIBER: 8G, SUGAR: 2G, PROTEIN: 8G

Beef Kabobs w/ tomato salad

Time: 40 minutes
Servings: 4-8

Ingredients

1 zucchini, quartered and chunked
4 mushrooms
½ pound sirloin, cut into 1 inch pieces
¼ cup prepared light Italian salad dressing

Marinade steak in dressing 5-30 minutes. Thread into skewers with vegetables. Grill 8 minutes. Pull from skewers and stuff into pita. Serve with Tomato Salad.

Nutritional Information (per serving)

CALORIES: 120, TOTAL FAT: 1G, SATURATED FAT: 0G, CHOLESTEROL: 0MG, SODIUM: 175MG, CARBOHYDRATES: 14G, FIBER: 8G, SUGAR: 2G, PROTEIN: 8G

 This recipe does not include nutritional information for the pita pocket bread. For this nutritional information, go to page 71.

Tomato Salad

Time: 5 minutes
Servings: 4

Ingredients
    2 tomatoes, seeded & chopped
    1 cucumber, peeled, seeded, & sliced
    ¼ red onion, thinly sliced
    2 T prepared light Italian salad dressing

Combine all ingredients in a small bowl

Nutritional Information (per serving)
CALORIES: 120, TOTAL FAT: 1G, SATURATED FAT: 0G, CHOLESTEROL: 0MG,
SODIUM: 175MG, CARBOHYDRATES: 14G, FIBER: 8G, SUGAR: 2G, PROTEIN: 8G

Asian Kabobs w/ Cucumber Salad

Time: 40 minutes
Servings: 4

Ingredients
    ½ pounds boneless skinless chicken breasts, cut into 1 inch pieces
    4 mushrooms
    4 asparagas, cut into 3 inch lengths
    4 scallions, cut into 3 inch lengths
    1 red pepper, chunked
    ¼ cup soy ginger dressing

Marinade chicken in dressing 5-30 minutes. Thread onto skewers alternating
with vegetables. Grill 8 minutes. Pull from the skewer and stuff into pita.
Serve with Cucumber Salad.

Nutritional Information (per serving)
CALORIES: 120, TOTAL FAT: 1G, SATURATED FAT: 0G, CHOLESTEROL: 0MG,
SODIUM: 175MG, CARBOHYDRATES: 14G, FIBER: 8G, SUGAR: 2G, PROTEIN: 8G

 This recipe does not include nutritional information for the pita
pocket bread. For this nutritional information, go to page 71.

Cucumber Salad

Time: 5 minutes
Servings: 4

Ingredients
    1 cucumber, peeled, seeded and thinly sliced
    1 carrot, grated
    3 T rice vinegar
    1 packet no-cal sweetener
    1 pinch red pepper flake
    1 T chopped peanuts

Combine all ingredients in a small bowl.

Nutritional Information (per serving)
CALORIES: 120, TOTAL FAT: 1G, SATURATED FAT: 0G, CHOLESTEROL: 0MG, SODIUM: 175MG, CARBOHYDRATES: 14G, FIBER: 8G, SUGAR: 2G, PROTEIN: 8G

Ham Kabobs

Time: 10 minutes
Servings: 4-8 skewers

Ingredients
    ½ pound ham, cut into 1 inch chunks
    1 can pineapple chunks, drained
    1 pepper, chunked
    4 cherry tomatoes
    ¼ cup teriyaki sauce

Toss all ingredients in teriyaki sauce and thread onto skewers. Grill 5 minutes. Pull from skewers and stuff into pita.

Nutritional Information (per serving)
CALORIES: 120, TOTAL FAT: 1G, SATURATED FAT: 0G, CHOLESTEROL: 0MG, SODIUM: 175MG, CARBOHYDRATES: 14G, FIBER: 8G, SUGAR: 2G, PROTEIN: 8G

 This recipe does not include nutritional information for the pita pocket bread. For this nutritional information, go to page 71.

Garden Kabobs

Time: 10 minutes
Servings: 4-8 skewers

Ingredients

4 mushrooms
1 pepper, chunked
1 zucchini, quartered & chunked
¼ onion, chunked
¼ cup prepared light Italian salad dressing

Toss all ingredients in dressing. Thread onto skewers. Grill 5 minutes. Pull from skewers and stuff into Pita.

Nutritional Information (per serving)

CALORIES: 120, TOTAL FAT: 1G, SATURATED FAT: 0G, CHOLESTEROL: 0MG, SODIUM: 175MG, CARBOHYDRATES: 14G, FIBER: 8G, SUGAR: 2G, PROTEIN: 8G

 This recipe does not include nutritional information for the pita pocket bread. For this nutritional information, go to page 71.

Tikka w/ Cucumber Raita

Time: 40 minutes
Servings: 4-8 skewers

Ingredients

1 pound boneless skinless chicken breasts, cut into 1 inch pieces
2 T plain non-fat yogurt
2 T tomato paste
½ onion, minced
2 T bottled minced garlic
1 T paprika
1/2 t ground ginger
¼ t salt
¼ t cumin
pinch cayenne
pinch nutmeg

In a small bowl combine all ingredients and allow to marinate at least 30 minutes. Thread onto skewers. Grill 8 minutes, or until chicken is cooked. Pull from the skewer and stuff into pita. Serve with Raita.

Nutritional Information (per serving)

CALORIES: 120, TOTAL FAT: 1G, SATURATED FAT: 0G, CHOLESTEROL: 0MG, SODIUM: 175MG, CARBOHYDRATES: 14G, FIBER: 8G, SUGAR: 2G, PROTEIN: 8G

 This recipe does not include nutritional information for the pita pocket bread. For this nutritional information, go to page 71.

Shrimp Kabobs

Time: 15 minutes
Servings: 4 – 8 skewers

Ingredients

½ pound large shrimp, peeled and deveined
¼ cup light Italian dressing
1 zucchini, quartered and chunked
4 mushrooms
4 cherry tomatoes
4 scallions, cut into 3 inch lengths

In a small bowl marinate shrimp in dressing. Thread onto skewers, alternating with vegetables. Grill 6 minutes, or until shrimp is cooked. Pull from the skewer and stuff into pita.

Nutritional Information (per serving)

CALORIES: 120, TOTAL FAT: 1G, SATURATED FAT: 0G, CHOLESTEROL: 0MG, SODIUM: 175MG, CARBOHYDRATES: 14G, FIBER: 8G, SUGAR: 2G, PROTEIN: 8G

 This recipe does not include nutritional information for the pita pocket bread. For this nutritional information, go to page 71.

mexican
pockets

Mexican Empanada

Time: 20
Servings: 4

Ingredients
½ pound boneless, skinless chicken breast, chopped
2 t pine nuts
3 stuffed green olives, chopped
½ t cumin
pinch red pepper flake
pinch cinnamon
2/3 cup onion, minced
1/3 cup raisins

Place a non-stick pan over medium heat and spray with cooking spray. Cook chopped chicken and onions until beginning to brown. Stir in remaining ingredients, cook 2 minutes, or until heated through. Fill pitas. If desired, serve with light sour cream.

Nutritional Information (per serving)
CALORIES: 100, TOTAL FAT: 2G, SATURATED FAT: 0G, CHOLESTEROL: 25MG, SODIUM: 85MG, CARBOHYDRATES: 11G, FIBER: 1G, SUGAR: 9G, PROTEIN: 9G

 This recipe does not include nutritional information for the pita pocket bread. For this nutritional information, go to page 71.

Sopapillas

Time: 10
Servings: 2

Ingredients
1 pita, divided into two rounds
1 T cinnamon sugar
1 t honey

Preheat oven to 425. Cut pita rounds into wedges. Arrange wedges on cookie sheet with sprayed with cooking spray. Mist tops of wedges with cooking spray. Dust with cinnamon sugar. Bake 4 minutes, or until crisp. Drizzle with honey & serve.

CALORIES: 50, TOTAL FAT: 0G, SATURATED FAT: 0G, CHOLESTEROL: 0MG, SODIUM: 70MG, CARBOHYDRATES: 12G, FIBER: 2G, SUGAR: 4G, PROTEIN: 2G

Nachos

Time: 10
Servings: 2

Ingredients

    1 pita, divided into two rounds
    ¼ cup non-fat refried beans (green chili & lime flavor)
    ¼ cup shredded cheese
    ¼ cup diced cooked chicken
    2 T minced onion
    1 T chopped cilantro
    2 T salsa
    1 T light sour cream

Preheat oven to 425. Cut pita rounds into wedges. Arrange wedges on cookie sheet with sprayed with cooking spray. Mist tops of wedges with cooking spray and bake 4 minutes, or until crisp. Top each wedge with a rounded teaspoon of beans, and a but of cheese, chicken , onion, cilantro and salsa. Return to the cookie sheet and bake until cheese melts, about a minute. Top each nacho with a dab of sour cream & serve.

Nutritional Information (per serving)

CALORIES: 170, TOTAL FAT: 6G, SATURATED FAT: 3.5G, CHOLESTEROL: 20MG, SODIUM: 460MG, CARBOHYDRATES: 19G, FIBER: 5G, SUGAR: 2G, PROTEIN: 9G

Tostadas

Time: 10
Servings: 2

Ingredients

    1 pita, divided into two rounds
    ½ cup non-fat refried beans (green chili & lime flavor)
    ¼ cup shredded cheese
    ¼ cup diced cooked chicken

2 T minced onion
1 T chopped cilantro
¼ cup shredded lettuce
2 T salsa
1 T light sour cream

Preheat oven to 425. Place pita rounds on a cooking sheet sprayed with cooking spray. Mist rounds with cooking spray and bake 4 minutes, or until crisp. Spread ¼ cup of beans over each tostada. Sprinkle cheese, chicken, onion, and cilantro evenly over both rounds. Return to the cookie sheet and bake until cheese melts, about a minute. Top each tostada with lettuce, salsa & sour cream & serve.

Nutritional Information (per serving)
CALORIES: 230, TOTAL FAT: 7G, SATURATED FAT: 4G, CHOLESTEROL: 55MG, SODIUM: 470MG, CARBOHYDRATES: 19G, FIBER: 5G, SUGAR: 3G, PROTEIN: 22G

Chicken Fajita

30

Time: 30 minutes
Servings: 6

Ingredients
3 skinless-split chicken breasts (12 oz. total)
1 green bell pepper; sliced into long strips
1 medium onion; sliced
1 T canola oil
1 t chicken fajita seasoning

Heat oil in large skillet on med-high heat for 1 minute. Season whole breast; sauté until brown (3-4 min. each side). Remove chicken from pan; slice into 1/2" x 1" strips. Add peppers and onions to pan; cook until tenders. Add chicken back to pan and stir with peppers & onion for 1-2 minutes. Fill pocket & serve.

Nutritional Information (per serving)
CALORIES: 125, TOTAL FAT: 4G, SATURATED FAT: 1G, CHOLESTEROL: 50MG, SODIUM: 152MG, CARBOHYDRATES: 3G, FIBER: 1G, SUGAR: 1G, PROTEIN: 18G

 This recipe does not include nutritional information for the pita pocket bread. For this nutritional information, go to page 71.

Beef Fajita

Time: 30 minutes
Servings: 6

Ingredients

12 oz. lean sirloin or beef tenderloin
1 green bell pepper; sliced into 1"strips
1 medium onion sliced
2 T canola oil
1 t beef fajita seasoning

Heat oil in large skillet on med-high heat for 1 minute. Season beef and sauté until browned (2-3 minute each side). Remove beef from pan; slice into thin 1" strips. Add peppers and onions to pan; cook until tender. Add beef back to pan; stir with peppers and onion for 1-2 minutes. Fill pocket & serve.

Nutritional Information (per serving)

CALORIES 214, TOTAL FAT 18G, SATURATED FAT 6G, CHOLESTEROL 40MG, SODIUM 152MG, CARBOHYDRATES 3G, FIBER 1G, SUGAR 1G, PROTEIN 10G

This recipe does not include nutritional information for the pita pocket bread. For this nutritional information, go to page 71.

peanut butter
pitas

Pocket Chef Jenna Says...

I am so glad the Pocket Diet book also focuses on children. So often overweight kids have their diets structured beyond belief, which only makes them sneak and rebel. It shows them to diet, not how to eat for the rest of their lives. The Pocket Diet teaches about portions and choices. You can eat what you like, but only a pocket's worth.

PBJ

Time: 5 minutes
Servings: 1

Ingredients
   1 T peanut butter
   1 T Sugar-free preserves (any flavor)
   1 pita half

Spread peanut butter inside one half of the pita. Spread preserves on the other half & serve.

Nutritional Information (per serving)
CALORIES: 150, TOTAL FAT: 8G, SATURATED FAT: 1.5G, CHOLESTEROL: 0MG, SODIUM: 90MG, CARBOHYDRATES: 18G, FIBER: 1G, SUGAR: 9G, PROTEIN: 4G

Grilled PBJ

Time: 5 minutes
Servings: 1

Ingredients
   1 T peanut butter
   1 T Sugar-free preserves (any flavor)
   1 pita half

Spread peanut butter inside one half of the pita. Spread preserves on the other half. Place a small non-stick skillet over medium high heat. Spray with butter flavor cooking spray. Grill one minute each side & serve.

Nutritional Information (per serving)
CALORIES: 160, TOTAL FAT: 8G, SATURATED FAT: 1.5G, CHOLESTEROL: 0MG, SODIUM: 90MG, CARBOHYDRATES: 18G, FIBER: 1G, SUGAR: 9G, PROTEIN: 4G

PB & Bacon

Time: 5 minutes
Servings: 1

Ingredients
1 T peanut butter
1 T reduced fat mayonnaise
1 lettuce leave
1 strip cooked bacon, halved (veggie bacon is fast and easy,
    a T of bacon bits works too)
1 pita half

Spread peanut butter inside one half of the pita. Spread mayonnaise on the other half. Arrange bacon and lettuce into pita & serve.

Nutritional Information (per serving)
CALORIES: 200, TOTAL FAT: 17G, SATURATED FAT: 5G, CHOLESTEROL: 20MG, SODIUM: 400MG, CARBOHYDRATES: 6G, FIBER: 1G, SUGAR: 2G, PROTEIN: 7G

Grilled Cheese & PB

Time: 5 minutes
Servings: 1

Ingredients
1 T peanut butter
1 slice reduced fat cheddar cheese
1 pita half

Spread peanut butter inside one half of the pita. Arrange cheese in pita. Place a small non-stick skillet over medium high heat. Spray with butter flavor cooking spray. Grill one minute each side, or until cheese melts & serve.

Nutritional Information (per serving)
CALORIES: 110, TOTAL FAT: 9G, SATURATED FAT: 2G, CHOLESTEROL: 5MG, SODIUM: 105MG, CARBOHYDRATES: 4G, FIBER: 1G, SUGAR: 1G, PROTEIN: 5G

PB & Applesauce

Time: 5 minutes
Servings: 1

Ingredients
  1 T peanut butter
  2 T Sugar-free applesauce
  1 pita half

Spread peanut butter inside one half of the pita. Spread applesauce on the other half & serve.

Nutritional Information (per serving)
CALORIES: 110, TOTAL FAT: 8G, SATURATED FAT: 1.5G, CHOLESTEROL: 0MG, SODIUM: 80MG, CARBOHYDRATES: 7G, FIBER: 1G, SUGAR: 4G, PROTEIN: 4G

PB & Apple

Time: 5 minutes
Servings: 1

Ingredients
  1 T peanut butter
  ¼ apple, sliced thin
  1 pita half

Spread peanut butter inside pita. Fill with apple slices & serve.

Nutritional Information (per serving)
CALORIES: 120, TOTAL FAT: 8G, SATURATED FAT: 1.5G, CHOLESTEROL: 0MG, SODIUM: 80MG, CARBOHYDRATES: 9G, FIBER: 2G, SUGAR: 5G, PROTEIN: 4G

FlufferNutter

....

Time: 5 minutes
Servings: 1

Ingredients
   1 T peanut butter
   1 T marshmallow cream
   1 pita half

Spread peanut butter inside one half of the pita. Spread marshmallow cream on the other half.

Nutritional Information (per serving)
CALORIES: 330, TOTAL FAT: 16G, SATURATED FAT: 5G, CHOLESTEROL: 80MG, SODIUM: 1550MG, CARBOHYDRATES: 22G, FIBER: 5G, SUGAR: 4G, PROTEIN: 21G

PB & Nutella

....

Time: 5 minutes
Servings: 1

Ingredients
   1 T peanut butter
   1 T Nutella (Chocolate hazelnut spread)
   1 pita half

Spread peanut butter inside one half of the pita. Spread Nutella on the other half.

Nutritional Information (per serving)
CALORIES: 160, TOTAL FAT: 8G, SATURATED FAT: 1.5G, CHOLESTEROL: 0MG, SODIUM: 90MG, CARBOHYDRATES: 19G, FIBER: 1G, SUGAR: 10G, PROTEIN: 4G

Peanut Butter & Banana

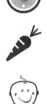

Time: 5 minutes
Servings: 2

Ingredients
    2 pita halves
    1/2 banana; sliced
    1 Tbsp. peanut butter; low fat
    1 Tsp. sugar-free fruit preserve (your choice)

Spread peanut butter in pocket. Add preserves, banana and serve.

Nutritional Information (per serving)
CALORIES: 225, TOTAL FAT: 6G, SATURATED FAT: 1G, CHOLESTEROL: 0MG, SODIUM: 95MG, CARBOHYDRATES: 45G, FIBER: 4G, SUGAR: 17G, PROTEIN: 7G

pita pie
pockets

Pocket Chef Jenna Says...

I've discovered a new way to warm pitas - upright in a loaf pan. Works in the microwave or oven, and keeps the stuffing from oozing out.

Apple Pie Pockets

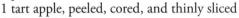

Time: 15 minutes
Servings: 2

Ingredients

2 pita halves
1 tart apple, peeled, cored, and thinly sliced
1 T apple juice
1 packet no calorie sweetener
1 t cinnamon
1 t cinnamon sugar

Preheat oven to 400. Place a non-stick pan over medium heat and spray with cooking spray. Add apple slices, juice, sweetener, and cinnamon. Cook until apple is tender, about 3 minutes. Spray outside of pitas with cooking spray. Sprinkle with cinnamon sugar. Set upright in a loaf pan. Divide apple filling between the two pockets. Bake 8 minutes, until filling is bubbly and pita is starting to brown.

Nutritional Information (per serving)
CALORIES: 130, TOTAL FAT: 0G, SATURATED FAT: 0G, CHOLESTEROL: 0MG, SODIUM: 140MG, CARBOHYDRATES: 29G, FIBER: 6G, SUGAR: 12G, PROTEIN: 3G

Cherry Pie Pockets

Time: 10 minutes
Servings: 2

Ingredients

2 pita halves
½ cup light cherry pie filling (mainly cherries)
1 t cinnamon sugar

Preheat oven to 400. Spray outside of pitas with cooking spray. Sprinkle with cinnamon sugar. Set upright in a loaf pan. Divide cherry filling between the two pockets. Bake 8 minutes, until filling is bubbly and pita is starting to brown.

Nutritional Information (per serving)
CALORIES: 160, TOTAL FAT: 0G, SATURATED FAT: 0G, CHOLESTEROL: 0MG, SODIUM: 150MG, CARBOHYDRATES: 37G, FIBER: 4G, SUGAR: 19G, PROTEIN: 3G

pita tarts

Pocket Chef Jenna Says...

Craving something decadent? How about something that tastes sinful...but isn't. Ever versatile pitas can be crisped into tart shells, and then topped with your favorite fruits. A guaranteed craving buster, that won't break your program. (If you can't find fruit flavored cream cheese, use an equal amount of light cream cheese and one packet no-cal sweetener)

Pita Tart Shell

Time: 5 minutes

Ingredients
 1 Pita half
 Cooking spray

Halve pita into two rounds. Place on a cookie sheet misted with cooking spray. Mist pitas with cooking spray. Bake at 400 for four minutes, or until crisp. Makes two shells. (If you crisp the pitas too long they may crumble when you slice the tart)

Fruit Tart

Time: 10 minutes
Servings: 1

Ingredients
 1 Pita Tart shell (see above)
 2 T seedless red grapes
 2 T seedless green grapes
 2 T blueberries, fresh or frozen
 3 T sugar-free apricot jam, divided

Spread 2 T jam into tart shell. Microwave remaining 1 T jam for 20 seconds. Toss fruit in melted jam and place in tart. Cut into wedges & serve.

Nutritional Information (per serving)
CALORIES: 130, TOTAL FAT: 0G, SATURATED FAT: 0G, CHOLESTEROL: 0MG, SODIUM: 140MG, CARBOHYDRATES: 30G, FIBER: 5G: SUGAR: 14G, PROTEIN: 3G

Raspberry Cream Tart

Time: 10 minutes
Servings: 1

Ingredients
1 Pita Tart shell (see page xx)
½ cup raspberries, fresh or frozen
¼ cup raspberry flavored whipped cream cheese

Spread cream cheese in tart shell. Top with raspberries. Cut into wedges & serve.

Nutritional Information (per serving)
CALORIES: 190, TOTAL FAT: 9G, SATURATED FAT: 6G, CHOLESTEROL: 30MG, SODIUM: 220MG, CARBOHYDRATES: 24G, FIBER: 8G, SUGAR: 5G, PROTEIN: 5G

Strawberry Cheesecake Tart

Time: 10 minutes
Servings: 1

Ingredients
1 Pita Tart shell (see page 204)
½ cup strawberries, sliced
¼ cup cheesecake flavored whipped cream cheese

Spread cream cheese in tart shell. Top with peach slices. Cut into wedges & serve.

Nutritional Information (per serving)
CALORIES: 210, TOTAL FAT: 11G, SATURATED FAT: 7G, CHOLESTEROL: 35MG, SODIUM: 240MG, CARBOHYDRATES: 22G, FIBER: 6G, SUGAR: 5G, PROTEIN: 6G

Chocolate Banana Tart

Time: 10 minutes
Servings: 1

Ingredients
1 Pita Tart shell
2 T chocolate chips, melted
1 banana sliced

Spread melted chocolate in tart shell (see page xx). Top with banana slices. Cut into wedges & serve.

Nutritional Information (per serving)

CALORIES: 300, TOTAL FAT: 7G, SATURATED FAT: 4G, CHOLESTEROL: 5MG, SODIUM: 160MG, CARBOHYDRATES: 56G, FIBER: 8G, SUGAR: 34G, PROTEIN: 6G

Peaches and Cream Tart

Time: 10 minutes
Servings: 1

Ingredients

1 Pita Tart shell (see page 204)
1 peach, sliced
¼ cup peach flavored whipped cream cheese

Spread cream cheese in tart shell. Top with peach slices. Cut into wedges & serve.

Nutritional Information (per serving)

CALORIES: 200, TOTAL FAT: 5G, SATURATED FAT: 3G, CHOLESTEROL: 20MG, SODIUM: 350MG, CARBOHYDRATES 29G, FIBER: 6G, SUGAR: 12G, PROTEIN: 10G

pizza
pockets

Pocket Chef Jenna Says...

Who doesn't love pizza? These can be made with any whole pita bread. Pocket-less pitas (flatbreads) are good if you like a chewier crust, but won't work for the double-decker pizza. Pasta sauce can be a little thin, making the pita-za crust soft. Our Pitza-Sauce, or any thick sauce, keeps the crust sliceable.

Pita-za Sauce

Time: 5 minutes
Servings: 2

Ingredients
   1 8oz can tomato paste
   1 t dried oregano
   ½ t garlic powder
   1 pinch crushed red pepper flake.

In a bowl combine all ingredients.

Nutritional Information (per serving)
CALORIES: 130, TOTAL FAT: 1G, SATURATED FAT: 0G, CHOLESTEROL: 0MG, SODIUM: 135MG, CARBOHYDRATES: 31G, FIBER: 7G, SUGAR: 4G, PROTEIN: 6G

Cheese Pita-za

Time: 10 minutes
Servings: 2

Ingredients
   1 pita
   2 T Pita-za sauce
   ¼ cup reduced-fat shredded mozzarella
   1 T grated parmesan

Spread sauce on pita. Sprinkle cheese over the sauce. Broil 5-7 minutes, until cheese is melted. Cut into 6 slices & serve.

(Use this as a base for your favorite toppings – pepperoni, onions, mushrooms, peppers, olives, jalapenos, pineapple, ham, etc.)

Nutritional Information (per serving)
CALORIES: 120, TOTAL FAT: 4.5G, SATURATED FAT: 3G, CHOLESTEROL: 15MG, SODIUM: 150MG, CARBOHYDRATES: 18G, FIBER: 4G, SUGAR: 1G, PROTEIN: 7G

Veggie Pita-za

Time: 10 minutes
Servings: 2

Ingredients

 1 pita
 2 T Pita-za sauce
 ¼ cup reduced-fat shredded mozzarella
 ¼ cup sliced mushrooms
 2 T red pepper, chopped
 1 T onion, minced

Spread sauce on pita. Sprinkle cheese over the sauce. Top with remaining ingredients. Broil 5-7 minutes, until cheese is melted. Cut into 6 slices & serve.

Nutritional Information (per serving)

CALORIES: 120, TOTAL FAT: 1G, SATURATED FAT: 0G, CHOLESTEROL: 0MG, SODIUM: 175MG, CARBOHYDRATES: 14G, FIBER: 8G, SUGAR: 2G, PROTEIN: 8G

BBQ Chicken Pita-za

Time: 10 minutes
Servings: 2

Ingredients

 1 pita
 2 T BBQ sauce
 2 T reduced-fat shredded cheddar
 2 T reduced-fat shredded mozzarella
 1 ounce cooked chicken, diced
 1 t cilantro leaves
 1 T red onions, chopped

Spread sauce on pita. Sprinkle cheese over the sauce. Top with remaining ingredients. Broil 5-7 minutes, until cheese is melted. Cut into 6 slices & serve.

Nutritional Information (per serving)

CALORIES: 130, TOTAL FAT: 1G, SATURATED FAT: 0G, CHOLESTEROL: 0MG, SODIUM: 135MG, CARBOHYDRATES: 31G, FIBER: 7G, SUGAR: 4G, PROTEIN: 6G

Cheeseburger Pita-za

Time: 10 minutes
Servings: 2

Ingredients
1 pita
2 T Pita-za sauce
¼ cup reduced-fat shredded cheddar
1 cooked hamburger patty, chopped

Spread sauce on pita. Sprinkle cheese over the sauce. Sprinkle hamburger over cheese. Broil 5-7 minutes, until cheese is melted. Cut into 6 slices & serve.

Nutritional Information (per serving)
CALORIES: 210. TOTAL FAT: 13G. SATURATED FAT: 6G, CHOLESTEROL: 50MG, SODIUM: 270MG, CARBOHYDRATES: 3G, FIBER: 7G, SUGAR: 2G, PROTEIN: 20G

Double Decker Pita-za

Time: 10 minutes
Servings: 2-3

Ingredients
1 pita pocket, split into two rounds
½ cup low-fat shredded mozzarella, divided
2 T Pita-za sauce
6 low fat pepperoni slices

Sprinkle one pita half with ¼ cup cheese. Top with remaining pita half. Spread with sauce. Sprinkle remaining cheese and arrange pepperoni slices. Broil 5-7 minutes, until cheese is melted. Cut into 6 slices & serve.

Nutritional Information (per serving)
CALORIES: 170, TOTAL FAT: 9G, SATURATED FAT: 4G, CHOLESTEROL: 20MG, SODIUM: 480MG, CARBOHYDRATES: 13G, FIBER: 1G, SUGAR: 1G, PROTEIN: 11G

Mexican Pita-za

Time: 10 minutes
Servings: 2

Ingredients

1 pita
¼ cup refried beans (non-fat, green chili & lime)
¼ cup reduced fat shredded cheddar
1 ounce cooked chicken, diced
1 t cilantro leaves
1 T frozen corn kernels
1 T onions, chopped
1 T salsa

Spread beans on pita. Sprinkle cheese over beans. Top with remaining ingredients. Broil 5-7 minutes, until cheese is melted. Cut into 6 slices & serve.

Nutritional Information (per serving)

CALORIES: 130, TOTAL FAT: 1.5, SATURATED FAT: .5G, CHOLESTEROL: 10MG, SODIUM: 340MG, CARBOHYDRATES: 19G, FIBER: 6G, SUGAR: 1G, PROTEIN: 8G

Margherita Pita-za

Time: 10 minutes
Servings: 2

Ingredients

1 pita
1 tomato, seeded and chopped
1 t bottled minced garlic
¼ cup reduced-fat shredded mozzarella
1 T grated parmesan
3 basil leaves, cut into thin strips

Scatter tomato and garlic over pita. Top with cheeses. Broil 5-7 minutes, until cheese is melted. Sprinkle basil over pita-za. Cut into 6 slices & serve.

Nutritional Information (per serving)

CALORIES: 200, TOTAL FAT: 5G, SATURATED FAT: 3G, CHOLESTEROL: 15MG, SODIUM: 330MG, CARBOHYDRATES: 27G, FIBER: 2G, SUGAR: 1G, PROTEIN: 12G

Pesto Pita-za

Time: 10 minutes
Servings: 2

Ingredients
1 pita
2 T reduced fat pesto
¼ cup reduced-fat shredded mozzarella
1 T grated parmesan
1 sundried tomato, chopped

Spread pesto over pita. Sprinkle with cheeses. Scatter tomato over the top. Broil 5-7 minutes, until cheese is melted. Cut into 6 slices & serve.

Nutritional Information (per serving)
CALORIES: 300, TOTAL FAT: 15G, SATURATED FAT: 5G, CHOLESTEROL: 20MG, SODIUM: 550MG, CARBOHYDRATES: 27G, FIBER: 2G, SUGAR: 2G, PROTEIN: 15G

Island Pita-za

Time: 10 minutes
Servings: 2

Ingredients
1 Pita
2 T bottled sweet and sour sauce
¼ cup reduced-fat shredded mozzarella
¼ cup chicken, cooked and chopped
1 green onion, chopped
¼ cup pineapple tidbits

Spread sauce on pita. Sprinkle cheese over sauce. Top with remaining ingredients. Broil 5-7 minutes, until cheese is melted. Cut into 6 slices & serve.

Nutritional Information (per serving)
CALORIES: 240, TOTAL FAT: 5G, SATURATED FAT: 2.5G, CHOLESTEROL: 30MG, SODIUM: 170MG, CARBOHYDRATES: 35G, FIBER: 7G, SUGAR: 23G, PROTEIN: 17G

Dessert Pita-za

Time: 10 minutes
Servings: 2

Ingredients

1 pita
1 tart apple, peeled, cored, and thinly sliced
1 T apple juice
1 packet no calorie sweetener
1 t cinnamon
¼ cup shredded reduced-fat cheddar

Place a non-stick pan over medium heat and spray with cooking spray. Add apple slices, juice, sweetener, and cinnamon. Cook until apple is tender, about 3 minutes. Arrange apples over pita. Sprinkle cheese on top. Broil 5-7 minutes, until cheese is melted. Cut into 6 slices & serve.

Nutritional Information (per serving)

CALORIES: 240, TOTAL FAT: 5G, SATURATED FAT: 3G, CHOLESTEROL: 15MG, SODIUM: 220MG, CARBOHYDRATES: 42G, FIBER: 6G, SUGAR: 13G, PROTEIN: 11G

pocket salads

Pocket Chef Jenna Says...

Salads are more than just lettuce and dressing. Jazz them up with bites of fruit, nuts, cheese, whatever strikes your fancy. Loaded with vegetables, fiber, and flavor, you're sure to be satisfied.

Strawberry Parmesan Salad

Time 5 minutes
Servings: 2

Ingredients

 1 cup romaine, shredded
 ¼ cup strawberries, sliced
 1 T red onion, diced
 1 T slivered almonds
 1 T parmesan cheese, grated
 1 T honey
 1 T balsamic vinegar

In a small bowl combine honey and vinegar. Toss in remaining ingredients. Fill pita & serve.

Nutritional Information (per serving)

CALORIES: 60, TOTAL FAT: 2G, SATURATED FAT: .5MG, CHOLESTEROL: 0MG, SODIUM: 40MG, CARBOHYDRATES: 109G, FIBER: 3, SUGAR: 8G, PROTEIN: 2G

 This recipe does not include nutritional information for the pita pocket bread. For this nutritional information, go to page 71.

Peach & Romaine Salad

Time: 5 minutes
Servings: 2

Ingredients

 1 cup romaine, shredded
 1 peach, sliced
 1 T red onion, diced
 1 T slivered almonds
 1 T blue cheese, crumbled
 1 T wine vinegar
 1 T olive oil

In a small bowl combine olive oil and vinegar. Toss in remaining ingredients. Fill pita & serve.

Nutritional Information (per serving)

CALORIES: 80, TOTAL FAT: 7G, SATURATED FAT: 1.5MG, CHOLESTEROL: 0MG, SODIUM: 110MG, CARBOHYDRATES: 5G, FIBER: 3, SUGAR: 4G, PROTEIN: 2G

 This recipe does not include nutritional information for the pita pocket bread. For this nutritional information, go to page 71.

Greek Salad

Time 5 minutes
Servings: 2

Ingredients

    1 cup romaine, shredded
    ¼ cup grape tomatoes
    ¼ cup cucumber, peeled, seeded, and diced
    1 T red onion, diced
    1 T feta cheese
    1 T wine vinegar
    1 T olive oil

In a small bowl combine olive oil and vinegar. Toss in remaining ingredients. Fill pita & serve.

Nutritional Information (per serving)

CALORIES: 90, TOTAL FAT: 3G, SATURATED FAT: 1.5MG, CHOLESTEROL: 00MG, SODIUM: 150MG, CARBOHYDRATES: 17G, FIBER: 5, SUGAR: 2G, PROTEIN: 3G

 This recipe does not include nutritional information for the pita pocket bread. For this nutritional information, go to page 71.

Spinach Salad

Time: 5 minutes
Servings: 2

Ingredients

    1 cup baby spinach leaves
    2 T lite balsamic vinaigrette
    ¼ cup sliced mushrooms
    1 T red onion, chopped
    1 slice bacon, crumbled

In a small bowl combine all ingredients. Fill pita & serve.

Nutritional Information (per serving)
CALORIES: 90, TOTAL FAT: 2G, SATURATED FAT: 1MG, CHOLESTEROL: 0MG, SODIUM: 150MG, CARBOHYDRATES: 5G, FIBER: 3, SUGAR: 4G, PROTEIN: 2G

 This recipe does not include nutritional information for the pita pocket bread. For this nutritional information, go to page 71.

Blue Cheese & Walnut Salad

Time: 5 minutes
Servings: 2

Ingredients
1 cup romaine, shredded
¼ cup red grapes, halved
1 T red onion, diced
¼ cup grape tomatoes
1 T blue cheese, crumbled
2 T walnuts, chopped
1 T balsamic vinegar
1 T olive oil.

In a small bowl combine olive oil and vinegar. Toss in remaining ingredients. Fill pita & serve.

Nutritional Information (per serving)
CALORIES: 100, TOTAL FAT: 8G, SATURATED FAT: 1.5MG, CHOLESTEROL: 0MG, SODIUM: 40MG, CARBOHYDRATES: 5G, FIBER: 3, SUGAR: 3G, PROTEIN: 2G

 This recipe does not include nutritional information for the pita pocket bread. For this nutritional information, go to page 71.

quesadilla
pockets

Pocket Chef Jenna Says...

Gooey, warm, and filled with flavor. Quesadillas make a great snack, or meal when paired with a simple salad tossed with dressing made from one part salsa and one part fat-free sour cream.

Steak Quesadillas

Time: 10 minutes
Servings: 2

Ingredients
    1 pita pocket, split into two rounds
    ½ cup grilled steak, diced
    1 T onion, minced
    1 T green pepper, minced
    ¼ cup reduced fat pepper jack cheese, shredded

Coat a non-stick skillet with cooking spray and place over medium-high heat. Place one pita half in pan, sprinkle with cheese, steak, peppers, and onion. Top with remaining pita half. Cook two minutes on each side, or until brown. Cut into wedges & serve.

Nutritional Information (per serving)
CALORIES: 320, TOTAL FAT: 23G, SATURATED FAT: 12G, CHOLESTEROL: 90MG, SODIUM: 480MG, CARBOHYDRATES: 4G, FIBER: 1G, SUGAR: 2G, PROTEIN: 24G

BBQ Chicken Quesadillas

Time: 10 minutes
Servings: 2

Ingredients
    1 pita pocket, split into two rounds
    ½ cup cooked chicken, diced
    1 T BBQ sauce
    1 T onion, minced
    1 T green pepper, minced
    ¼ cup reduced fat Monterey Jack cheese, shredded

In a small bowl stir cooked chicken in to BBQ sauce. Coat a non-stick skillet with cooking spray and place over medium-high heat. Place one pita half in pan, sprinkle with cheese, chicken, peppers, and onion. Top with remaining pita half. Cook two minutes on each side, or until brown. Cut into wedges & serve.

Nutritional Information (per serving)
CALORIES: 120, TOTAL FAT: 4G, SATURATED FAT: 1G, CHOLESTEROL: 35MG, SODIUM: 500MG, CARBOHYDRATES: 3G, FIBER: 1G, SUGAR: 3G, PROTEIN: 16G

Krab Quesadillas

Time: 10 minutes
Servings: 2

Ingredients
    1 pita pocket, split into two rounds
    ½ cup imitation crab (krab), diced
    1 T frozen corn kernels, thawed
    1 T red pepper, minced
    ¼ cup reduced fat Monterey Jack cheese, shredded

In a small bowl stir cooked chicken in to BBQ sauce. Coat a non-stick skillet with cooking spray and place over medium-high heat. Place one pita half in pan, sprinkle with cheese, krab, peppers, and corn. Top with remaining pita half. Cook two minutes on each side, or until brown. Cut into wedges & serve.

Nutritional Information (per serving)
CALORIES: 150, TOTAL FAT: 5G, SATURATED FAT: 3.5G, CHOLESTEROL: 45MG, SODIUM: 700MG, CARBOHYDRATES: 8G, FIBER: 0G, SUGAR: 5G, PROTEIN: 17G

shrimp

Shrimp Scampi

Time: 10 minutes
Servings: 2-3

Ingredients

1 t extra virgin olive oil
1 t butter
1 garlic clove, minced
½ pound peeled, deveined shrimp
¼ cup sliced mushrooms
½ cup white wine
1 t chopped parsley
1 T lemon juice

In a pan, heat oil and butter over medium high heat. Add garlic shrimp and mushrooms. Cook 2 minutes. Flip shrimp over and add wine, parsley, and lemon juice. Cook until almost dry. Fill pitas & serve.

Nutritional Information (per serving)

CALORIES: 200, TOTAL FAT: 6G, SATURATED FAT: 2G, CHOLESTEROL: 225MG, SODIUM: 280MG, CARBOHYDRATES: 3G, FIBER: 2G, SUGAR: 1G, PROTEIN: 24G

 This recipe does not include nutritional information for the pita pocket bread. For this nutritional information, go to page 71.

Southern Shrimp

Time: 10 minutes
Servings: 2-3

Ingredients

1 t butter
1 t bacon bits
1 garlic clove, minced
½ pound peeled, deveined shrimp
¼ cup sliced mushrooms
1 green onion, sliced
1 dash hot pepper sauce
1 t chopped parsley
1 T lemon juice

In a pan, butter over medium high heat. Add bacon bits, garlic, shrimp, and mushrooms. Cook 2 minutes. Flip shrimp over and add green onion, hot pepper sauce, parsley, and lemon juice. Cook until almost dry. Fill pitas & serve.

Nutritional Information (per serving)
CALORIES: 150, TOTAL FAT: 4G, SATURATED FAT: 1.5G, CHOLESTEROL: 180MG, SODIUM: 230MG, CARBOHYDRATES: 4G, FIBER: 0G, SUGAR: 1G, PROTEIN: 24G

 This recipe does not include nutritional information for the pita pocket bread. For this nutritional information, go to page 71.

Shrimp Po' Boy

Time: 15 minutes
Servings: 2

Ingredients
8 battered frozen shrimp, baked
2 T ketchup
1 T lemon juice
1 shake worcesterchire sauce
1 shake hot sauce
2 lettuce leaves
2 red onion slices
2 pita pockets (1/2 each)

In a small bowl combine ketchup, lemon juice, Worcestershire, and hot sauce to make a spicy mix. Spread inside pitas. Arrange shrimp, lettuce & onions in pitas & serve.

Nutritional Information (per serving)
CALORIES: 250, TOTAL FAT: 6G, SATURATED FAT: 1G, CHOLESTEROL: 30MG, SODIUM: 630MG, CARBOHYDRATES: 39G, FIBER: 6G, SUGAR: 7G, PROTEIN: 11G

Dill Shrimp

Time: 15 minutes
Servings: 10

Ingredients
2 lbs. cooked shrimp (small or medium size)
3 scallions; chopped

2 celery stalks; chopped
¼ cup plain yogurt; low fat
¼ cup mayonnaise; low fat
1 T fresh dill; chopped
2 lemons; juiced
1 lime; juiced

Combine all ingredients in large bowl and mix well. Refrigerate until chilled. Fill pocket & serve.

Nutritional Information (per serving)

CALORIES: 76, TOTAL FAT: 1G, SATURATED FAT: 0G, CHOLESTEROL: 2MG, SODIUM: 476MG, CARBOHYDRATES: 5G, FIBER: 2G, SUGAR: 1G, PROTEIN: 12G

 This recipe does not include nutritional information for the pita pocket bread. For this nutritional information, go to page 71.

Shrimp & Avocado

Time: 15 minutes
Servings: 8

Ingredients

1 lb. cooked shrimp; rinse & dry (small or medium size)
2 avocados; diced
3 T olive oil
2 medium garlic cloves; minced
2 T cilantro; chopped
2 T lime juice
1 t ground cumin
1 t jalapeno sauce (optional)

Whisk limejuice, garlic, cumin, olive oil, jalapeno sauce and cilantro. Place avocado in mixture; let marinate for 5 minutes. Salt & pepper to taste. Fill pocket & serve.

Nutritional Information (per serving)

CALORIES: 140, TOTAL FAT: 11G, SATURATED FAT: 1G, CHOLESTEROL: 2MG SODIUM: 278MG, CARBOHYDRATES: 4G, FIBER: 2G, SUGAR: 0G, PROTEIN: 9G

 This recipe does not include nutritional information for the pita pocket bread. For this nutritional information, go to page 71.

Spicy Shrimp Salad

Time: 5 minutes
Servings: 2-4

Ingredients

½ pound cooked salad shrimp
¼ cup light mayonnaise
1 t lemon juice
1 t tomato paste
1 t prepared horseradish
2 shakes Worcestershire
1 shake Tabasco
1 pinch sugar

In a small bowl combine all ingredients. Fill pitas & serve.

Nutritional Information (per serving)

CALORIES: 140, TOTAL FAT: 7G, SATURATED FAT: 1.5G, CHOLESTEROL: 145MG, SODIUM: 320MG, CARBOHYDRATES: 2G, FIBER: 0G, SUGAR: 0G, PROTEIN: 16G

take out inspired

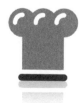 ## *Pocket Chef Jenna Says...*

There are days when there is no time to prepare a complete meal, hence why so many of us hit the drive through. But, minute for minute these options are faster, not to mention much cheaper. If you have a child interested in the program, these will be instant favorites.

Egg McPita

Time: 5 minutes
Servings: 1

Ingredients
1 pita half
1 egg
1 slice reduced fat American cheese
1 slice turkey ham lunchmeat

Heat a small non-stick pan over medium-high heat. Spray with cooking spray and crack egg into pan. Cook until bottom is set, about 1 minute, then flip and cook until desired doneness. Arrange in pita with ham & cheese.

Nutritional Information (per serving)
CALORIES: 280, TOTAL FAT: 13G, SATURATED FAT: 6G, CHOLESTEROL: 305MG, SODIUM: 750MG, CARBOHYDRATES: 18G, FIBER: 4G, SUGAR: 3G, PROTEIN: 21G

Fish Stick Pita

Time: 5 minutes
Servings: 2

Ingredients
1 pita half
3 fish sticks, heated
1 slice reduced fat American cheese
1 T fat free tartar sauce
¼ cup shredded lettuce

Spread inside of pita with Tartar sauce. Stuff with remaining ingredients & serve.

Nutritional Information (per serving)
CALORIES: 400, TOTAL FAT: 17G, SATURATED FAT: 7G, CHOLESTEROL: 115MG, SODIUM: 1040MG, CARBOHYDRATES: 39G, FIBER: 5G, SUGAR: 3G, PROTEIN: 21G

Club House Pita

5

Time: 5 minutes
Servings: 2

Ingredients

1 pita half
1 slice turkey lunch meat
1 slice ham lunchmeat
1 T reduced-fat mayo
1 slice reduced fat cheddar
2 tomato slices
1 T BBQ sauce

Inside the pita, spread half with mayo, half with BBQ sauce. Arrange the meat, cheese, and tomato inside. Grill (or microwave if you are at work) in a nonstick pan coated with cooking spray until cheese melts.

Nutritional Information (per serving)

CALORIES: 220, TOTAL FAT: 5G, SATURATED FAT: 2.5G, CHOLESTEROL: 35MG, SODIUM: 1000MG, CARBOHYDRATES: 26G, FIBER: 4G, SUGAR: 8G, PROTEIN: 16G

The Pocket Diet & Recipe Book

tuna
pockets

Pocket Chef Jenna Says...

Tuna in a can or fresh is healthy for the heart and will leave your taste buds satisfied.

Traditional Tuna Salad

Time: 5 minutes
Servings: 2

Ingredients

  2 pita halves
  1 can water packed tuna, well drained
  2 T light mayonnaise
  1 T sweet pickle relish
  Salt & Pepper to taste to taste

Mix ingredients in a small bowl. Fill pita & serve.

Nutritional Information (per serving)
CALORIES: 170, TOTAL FAT: 8G, SATURATED FAT: 1.5G, CHOLESTEROL: 35MG,
SODIUM: 1090MG, CARBOHYDRATES: 4G, FIBER: 0G, SUGAR: 2G, PROTEIN: 20G

Twisted Tuna Salad

Time: 5 minutes
Servings: 2

Ingredients

  2 pita halves
  1 can water packed tuna, well drained
  Juice of half a lemon (twist of lemon)
  2 T light mayonnaise
  1 T dill pickle relish
  1 stalk of celery, diced
  Salt & Pepper to taste

Mix ingredients in a small bowl. Fill pita and serve.

Nutritional Information (per serving)
CALORIES: 180, TOTAL FAT: 8G, SATURATED FAT: 1.5G, CHOLESTEROL: 35MG,
SODIUM: 1090MG, CARBOHYDRATES: 6G, FIBER: 0G, SUGAR: 3G, PROTEIN: 20G

Tuna Salad Supreme

Time: 5 minutes
Servings: 4

Ingredients
4 pita halves
6 oz. albacore white tuna in water; drained
1/4 cup celery; diced
1/4 cup pickles; diced (or relish)
1/4 cup apple; diced
1/4 cup onion diced
3 T mayonnaise; low fat
1 t horseradish

Mix all ingredients in a small bowl. Salt & pepper to taste. Fill pocket & serve.

Nutritional Information (per serving)
CALORIES: 84, TOTAL FAT: 2G, SATURATED FAT: 0G, CHOLESTEROL: 20MG, SODIUM: 398MG, CARBOHYDRATES: 6G, FIBER: 1G, SUGAR: 2G, PROTEIN: 10G

Tuna Tarragon Salad

Time: 5 minutes
Servings: 2

Ingredients
2 pita halves
1 can water packed tuna, well drained
2 T light mayonnaise
1 T sweet pickle relish
1 T sweet pickle juice
1 stalk of celery, diced
1 T fresh tarragon, chopped
Salt & Pepper to taste

Mix ingredients in a small bowl. Fill pita and serve.

Nutritional Information (per serving)
CALORIES: 170, TOTAL FAT: 8G, SATURATED FAT: 1.5G, CHOLESTEROL: 35MG, SODIUM: 630MG, CARBOHYDRATES: 3G, FIBER: 8G, SUGAR: 1G, PROTEIN: 21G

Fancy Pants Tuna Salad

Time: 5 minutes
Servings: 2

Ingredients
  2 pita halves
  1 can water packed tuna, well drained
  1 T light mayonnaise
  1 T light sour cream
  1 green onion, chopped
  1 stalk of celery, chopped
  4 green olives, chopped
  1 T capers
  1 shake Worcestershire sauce

Mix ingredients in a small bowl. Fill pita and serve.

Nutritional Information (per serving)
CALORIES: 230, TOTAL FAT: 7G, SATURATED FAT: 2G, CHOLESTEROL: 40MG, SODIUM: 790MG, CARBOHYDRATES: 17G, FIBER: 8G, SUGAR: 8G, PROTEIN: 21G

Crunchy Tuna Salad

Time: 5 minutes
Servings 2

Ingredients
  2 pita halves
  1 can water packed tuna, well drained
  2 T light mayonnaise
  1 stalk of celery, diced
  ¼ cup water chestnuts, chopped
  1 green onion, chopped
  1 t soy sauce

Mix ingredients in a small bowl. Fill pita and serve.

Nutritional Information (per serving)
CALORIES: 250, TOTAL FAT: 8G, SATURATED FAT: 1.5G, CHOLESTEROL: 35MG, SODIUM: 710MG, CARBOHYDRATES: 19G, FIBER: 8G, SUGAR: 8G, PROTEIN: 21G

Tangy Tuna Salad

Time: 5 minutes
Servings 2

Ingredients
    2 pita halves
    1 can water packed tuna, well drained
    2 T light mayonnaise
    1/4 cup bottled pickled vegetables, drained and chopped
    2 T red onion, chopped
    Salt & Pepper to taste

Mix ingredients in a small bowl. Fill pita and serve.

Nutritional Information (per serving)
CALORIES: 170, TOTAL FAT: 8G, SATURATED FAT: 1.5G, CHOLESTEROL: 35MG, SODIUM: 630MG, CARBOHYDRATES: 3G, FIBER: 0G, SUGAR: 1G, PROTEIN: 21G

Orange Tuna Salad

Time: 5 minutes
Servings: 2

Ingredients
    2 pita halves
    1 can water packed tuna, well drained
    2 T light mayonnaise
    ¼ cup canned mandarin orange segments, drained
    2 T cashews, chopped
    ½ t ground ginger
    Salt & Pepper to taste

Mix ingredients in a small bowl. Fill pita and serve.

Nutritional Information (per serving)
CALORIES: 220, TOTAL FAT: 12G, SATURATED FAT: 2.5G, CHOLESTEROL: 35MG, SODIUM: 490MG, CARBOHYDRATES: 6G, FIBER: 0G, SUGAR: 3G, PROTEIN: 22G

Herb Tuna Salad

Time: 5 minutes
Servings: 2

Ingredients

2 pita halves
1 can water packed tuna, well drained
1 T light mayonnaise
1 T fat-free, plain yogurt
1 T chives, snipped
1 T dill, chopped
1 T parsley, chopped
1 stalk of celery, diced
Salt & Pepper to taste

Mix ingredients in a small bowl. Fill pita and serve.

Nutritional Information (per serving)

CALORIES: 150, TOTAL FAT: 5G, SATURATED FAT: 1G, CHOLESTEROL: 35MG, SODIUM: 1280MG, CARBOHYDRATES: 3G, FIBER: 0G, SUGAR: 1G, PROTEIN: 21G

Mexican Tuna Salad

Time: 5 minutes
Servings: 2

Ingredients

2 pita halves
1 can water packed tuna, well drained
2 T salsa
2 T light sour cream
1 green onion, chopped
1 stalk of celery, chopped
½ t cumin
Salt & Pepper to taste.

Mix ingredients in a small bowl. Fill pita and serve.

Nutritional Information (per serving)

CALORIES: 210, TOTAL FAT: 4G, SATURATED FAT: 1.5G, CHOLESTEROL: 40MG, SODIUM: 1370MG, CARBOHYDRATES: 18G, FIBER: 8G, SUGAR: 10G, PROTEIN: 22G

Cheesy Tuna Salad

Time: 5 minutes
Servings: 2

Ingredients

2 pita halves
1 can water packed tuna, well drained
1 T light mayonnaise
¼ cup low-fat cottage cheese
2 T reduced-fat sharp cheddar cheese, grated
1 T parmesan cheese, grated
1 green onion, chopped
1 stalk of celery, chopped
Salt & Pepper to taste

Mix ingredients in a small bowl. Fill pita and serve.

Nutritional Information (per serving)

CALORIES: 290, TOTAL FAT: 9G, SATURATED FAT: 3.5G, CHOLESTEROL: 50MG, SODIUM: 1580MG, CARBOHYDRATES: 17G, FIBER: 8G, SUGAR: 8G, PROTEIN: 30G

Apple Walnut Tuna

Time: 15 minutes
Servings: 2

Ingredients

2 pita halves
6 oz albacore tuna (in water); drained
1/4 cup celery; diced
1/4 cup walnuts; chopped
1 med. apple; diced
3 T mayonnaise; low fat
1 T dijon mustard
1 T sweet pickle relish

Combine all ingredients in a small bowl. Salt & pepper to taste. Fill pocket & serve.

Nutritional Information (per serving)

CALORIES: 150, TOTAL FAT: 7G, SATURATED FAT: 1G, CHOLESTEROL: 20MG, SODIUM: 378MG, CARBOHYDRATES: 11G, FIBER: 2G, SUGAR: 6G, PROTEIN: 11G

Tuna & Cannellini Salad

Time: 5 minutes
Servings: 6-8

Ingredients

1 15 oz can cannelloni beans, drained & rinsed
1 6 oz can tuna in olive oil
¼ cup red onion, diced
1 T red wine vinegar
1 T parsley, chopped
salt and pepper

In a large bowl combine all ingredients. Fill pitas & serve.

Nutritional Information (per serving)

CALORIES: 120, TOTAL FAT: 5G, SATURATED FAT: 1G, CHOLESTEROL: 15MG, SODIUM: 250MG, CARBOHYDRATES: 10G, FIBER: 3G, SUGAR: 2G, PROTEIN: 8G

 This recipe does not include nutritional information for the pita pocket bread. For this nutritional information, go to page 71.

Appendix

- Free Foods
- Foods High in Saturated & Trans-Fats
- Vegetables Non-Starch & High Starch
- Heart Healthy Proteins
- Milk Substitutes
- Pocket Bread Equivalents

Free Food List

A free food is any food or drink that contains less than 20 calories per serving. No more than 2-3 servings of these foods (with correlated portion size) should be eaten in one day, otherwise the calories of each item must be included as part of the food servings allowed in your diet plan.

Fat-Free or Reduced Fat	Serving Size
Cream cheese, fat free	1 Tbsp.
Creamers, non-dairy, liquid	1 Tbsp.
Creamers, non dairy, powder	2 tsp.
Mayonnaise fat free	1 Tbsp.
Mayonnaise, reduced fat	1 tsp.
Miracle whip, fat-free	1 Tbsp.
Miracle whip, reduced fat	1tsp.
Salad dressing, fat free or low fat	2 Tbsp.
Sour cream, fat free or reduced fat	1 Tbsp.
Non stick cooking spray	Unlimited

Sugar Free Foods	Serving Size
Jam or jelly, light	2 tsp.
Syrup, sugar free	2 Tbsp.
Candy, hard, sugar free	1 candy
Gelatin dessert, sugar free	Unlimited
Gelatin, unflavored	Unlimited
Gum, sugar free	Unlimited
Sugar substitutes	Unlimited

Liquids	Serving Size
Cocoa powder, unsweetened	1 Tbsp.
Bouillon, broth, consommé	Unlimited
Carbonated, mineral, tonic water	Unlimited
Coffee	Unlimited
Drink mixes, sugar free	Unlimited
Tea, caffeine and sugar free	Unlimited

Condiments Serving Size	
Ketchup, mustard, horseradish, relish	1 Tbsp.
Lime juice, lemon juice	1 Tbsp.
Pickle, dill (medium)	1 1/2
Salsa	1/4 cup.
Taco sauce	1 Tbsp.
Soy sauce, regular or light	1 Tbsp.
Flavoring extracts, garlic, herbs, spices	Unlimited
Tabasco, cooking wine, Worcestershire	Unlimited

Food High In Saturated & Trans-Fats

Saturated Fats: Fats found in animal products.

Meats

Goose, duck, poultry skin, giblets
Organ meat (liver, kidney)
Hot dogs, sausage or bacon

Dairy

Whole milk
Whole milk yogurt, pudding
Evaporated whole milk
High fat cheeses
Ice Cream

Fats & Oils

Lard, butter, palm oil, kernel oil, beef tallow, cocoa butter,
coconut oil, salt pork

Trans-Fats: Foods made with hydrogenated oil.
These foods typically contain hydrogenated or partially hydrogenated oil.
We recommend that you read the label.

Cake mixes, biscuit, pancake and cornbread mixes, frostings

Cakes, cookies, muffins, pies, donuts

Crackers

Peanut butter (except fresh-ground)

Frozen entrees and meals

Frozen bakery products, toaster pastries, waffles, pancakes

Most prepared frozen meats and fish (such as fish sticks)

French fries

Whipped toppings

Margarines, shortening

Instant mashed potatoes

Taco shells

Cocoa mix

Microwave popcorn

Non-starchy Vegetables

These vegetables contain high complex carbohydrates and they are loaded with nutrients and fibers. Eat these vegetables in abundance as snacks or with meals. (1 serving = 1 cup raw or 1/2 cup cooked or juiced)

Artichoke	Eggplant	Salad greens
Asparagus	Green Onions, scallions	Sauerkraut
Beans (green, wax, italian)	Kohlrabi	Spinach
Bean sprouts	Leeks	Summer squash
Beets	Mixed vegetables	Tomato, fresh
Broccoli	(without corn, peas	Turnips
Brussels Sprouts	or pasta)	Water chestnuts
Cabbage	Mushrooms	Zucchini
Carrots	Onions	
Cauliflower	Pea Pods	
Celery	Peppers (all varieties)	
Cucumber	Radishes	

Heart Healthy Proteins

- Dried beans (legumes) and peas
- Lamb: leg, loin chop, sirloin, poultry, beef tenderloin, lean beef
- Pork: tenderloin, pork loin, ham, loin chops, Canadian bacon
- Veal: loin chop, sirloin, cutlet, ground
- Venison, rabbit, buffalo, ostrich
- Reduced fat lunch meats, (less than 5 grams of fat per ounce)
- Cheese & cottage cheese (less than 3-5 grams of fat per ounce)
- Egg whites
- Tofu

Milk Substitutes

(For those who do not like milk or cannot drink it for health reasons)
1 cup of milk is equivalent to:

Yogurt, low fat, fat free	3/4 cup	Low fat frozen yogurt	1/2 cup
Cottage cheese, low fat	3/4 cup	Calcium fortified juice	3/4 cup
Low fat cheese, hard	1 1/2 ounce slice	Low fat pudding	1/2 cup
		Fortified soy milk	1 cup

Pocket Bread Equivalent

One Kangaroo Pocket is: White = 90 calories • Wheat = 80 calories

Use this as a guide when substituting any of these foods for a pocket bread.

Equivalent To	Serving Size
Traditional loaf Bread	1 slice
English muffin	1/2
Hot dog or Hamburger bun	1/2
Small Roll, plain	1
6" Tortilla (corn & flour)	1
Bran cereal	1/2 cup
Granola, low fat	1/4 cup
Grape nuts	1/4 cup
Pasta	1/3 cup
Puffed cereal	1 1/2 cups
Rice	1/3 cup
Wheat germ	3 Tbsp.
Waffle, reduced fat	1
Baked beans	1/3 cup
Corn	1/2 cup
Corn on cob	1/2 cob
Mixed veggies	1 cup
Green Peas	1/2 cup
Potato, boiled or mashed	1/2 cup
Squash, winter	1 cup
Yam, sweet potato	1/2 cup
Graham crackers	3
Popcorn, no fat	3 cups
Rice cakes	2
Saltine Crackers	6
Potato chips, baked, fat free	15-20

Here is what Pocket Diet users are saying...

"The Pocket Diet is easy to follow, fun & rewarding! I realized I could lose weight without starving myself. I used to skip breakfast and ate very little lunch. Now I can eat three meals & still lose weight. It's wonderful."

Anne L. — Sussex, WI

"My wife and I both started last Monday and we were thrilled that when we weighed this morning we had both lost 5 pounds. I have also started walking according to the e-Plan Walking Program... 2 miles each day but this morning I got brave and walked 3.25 miles. Having been on many other diets through the years, we are finding that his is the best we have tried."

AJ — Arkansas

"I got the bread I craved and quick results – down nine pounds in my first week and 100 pounds in 15 months. I love my size-6 jeans. They're so small!"

Kathy Y. — Myrtle Beach, SC

"I can't begin to thank you enough for the effort you have taken to produce a sound, easy and nutritious way to lose excess pounds. The results I have achieved on the Pocket Diet so far are an amazing 17 pound loss and two pant sizes in 6 weeks! Believe me when I tell you I wish I had heard about this diet long before now. I have struggled with yo-yo dieting for many years to only lose weight, regain and add extra pounds back. This is the easiest diet to follow. To those who are considering trying this diet I say, you will be amazed at the ease and how successful you will be."

Suzette K.

"Until I started the Pocket Diet, I never ate breakfast...I would have my cup of coffee and that was it. The pita pockets make it so easy to just scramble up an egg or cut up some fruit, put it in the pocket and you are out the door. There is barely any cleanup and they're easy-to-eat on the road. The pockets are excellent for helping determine portion sizes, which is something that I've never watched in the past. I really like this diet because there are so many tasty recipes to choose from."

Lisa B. — North Prairie, WI

"We barely ever buy bread in our household. The pita pockets help control
portion size and I love the way they taste. My teenager even likes them."

Anita B. — Menomonee Fall, WI

"I have been on the diet for 5 weeks and have lost 14 pounds and my husband has lost 14 1/2 pounds. My biggest problem with other diets is that I love carbs and other diets severely limit them. So being able to have bread at every meal is wonderful!! I feel absolutely filled up and for the first time in my memory and not craving sweets."

Pat J. — Bella Vista, AR

"I lost 11 pounds the first 3 weeks...but my husband has now surpassed me with ongoing weight loss, at an amazing speed. With 5 weeks down I have lost 12 pounds, ...and he has lost 22!"

PJ — Michigan

"In two and a half weeks, I was down 11 pounds. This is the best '"diet'" I have ever tried. It's easy and you don't have to buy special foods."

Nancy — Ohio

For more information, visit:

www.pocketdiet.com

Recipes
Menu Plans
Free Newsletter
Pocket News
Downloadable ePlans
Pocket Chat
Message Board
Diet & Fitness Tips
Team Competitions
Success Stories
Pocket Buddies
Contests & Special Promotions
Shopping
Diet Support
And more...

*Be sure to tell you friends
and family about*

The Pocket Diet!

The Pocket Diet & Recipe Book